WORKBOOK TO ACCOMPANY

MOSBY'S

Canadian
Textbook

FOR THE

Support Worker

ART 1029

0917-544/040

MOSBY'S
Canadian
Textbook
FOR THE
Support Worker

RELDA TIMMENY KELLY, RN, BSN, MSN
Instructor
Kankalee Community College

SHEILA A. SORRENTINO, RN, PHD
Curriculum and Health Care Consultant
Normal, Illinois

ROSEMARY GOODACRE, RN
Instructor and Co-ordinator, Personal Support Worker Program
Fleming College

N꤮ Mosby

National Library of Canada Cataloguing in Publication

Kelly, Relda Timmeney
    The workbook to accompany Mosby's Canadian textbook for the support worker /
Relda Timmeny Kelly; Canadian editor, Rosemary Goodacre.

ISBN 0-7796-9964-5

    1. Nurses' aides—Problems, exercises, etc. I. Goodacre, Rosemary. II. Sorrentino, Sheila A.
Mosby's Canadian textbook for the support worker. III. Title.

RT84.S67 2003 Suppl.   610.73'06'98   C2003-907188-X

Acquisitions Editor: Ann Millar
Editorial Manager: Zak Knowles
Developmental Editor: Lise Creurer
Publishing Services Manager: Gayle May
Production Manager: Joseph Selby
Designer: Kathi Gosche
Printing and binding: Courier

Elsevier Canada
1 Goldthorne Ave., Toronto, ON, Canada M8Z 5S7
Phone: 1-866-896-3331
Fax: 1-866-359-9534

Printed in the United States of America.

2 3 4 5   07 06 05 04

To Earl, my best friend and husband.
Without his support and encouragement
(as well as patience in eating many fast food meals),
I would have found this project impossible.

To my daughter, Elisabeth, who helped in so many little ways
to lessen the load on days when I faltered.

To my grandson, Samuel,
who provides joy and laughter every day.

To my friends Cindy, Helen, and Patty
for providing loads of love and moral support.

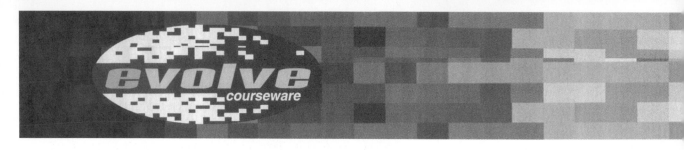

The Latest *Evolution* in Learning.

Evolve provides online access to free learning resources and activities designed specifically for the textbook you are using in your class. The resources will provide you with information that enhances the material covered in this book and much more.

Visit the Web address listed below to start your learning evolution today!

 LOGIN: *http://evolve.elsevier.com/Canada/Sorrentino/SupportWorker*

Evolve Online Courseware for Sorrentino: *Mosby's Canadian Textbook for the Support Worker* offers the following features:

● **Content Updates**
New and updated information related to this textbook.

● **Additional Resources**
Additional materials to enhance textbook content.

● **Links to Related Websites**
Links to other sites related to content in this textbook.

● **Links to Related Products**
See what else Elsevier Science has to offer in a specific field of interest.

Think outside the book . . . evolve

CREDITS AND REVIEWERS

ILLUSTRATION CREDITS

p. 200, unnumbered figure: Courtesy Laurel Wiersema-Bryant, RN, MSN, Clinical Nurse Specialist, Barnes-Jewish Hospital, St. Louis.

CANADIAN REVIEWER

Judith Bowyer, BScN, MEd
The Bowyer Group, Inc.
Toronto, Ontario

REVIEWERS

Donna Albrothross, RN, BSN
Registered Nurse
Loch Haven Nursing Home
Macon, Missouri

Beverly Sigl Felton, RN, MS, CS, ANP
Advanced Practice Nurse Prescriber
Gero-Psych Nursing, SC
Lannon, Wisconsin

Jana Gilbertson, RN, CDONA
Group Medical Services Manager
Beverly Healthcare
Louisville, Kentucky

Judy Kramer, RN, BSN, BS
San Clemente, California

June Edwards, RN
In-service Coordinator/Restorative Nurse
BHCC
Bridgton, Maine

INTRODUCTION

This workbook is intended to be used with *Mosby's Canadian Textbook for the Support Worker.* Additional resources are not required to complete the exercises in this workbook.

The workbook is designed as a study guide to help you apply what you have learned in each chapter of the textbook. A variety of learning exercises are presented and independent learning activities can be used to apply information in each chapter to individual situations. Supplementary to this workbook, procedure checklists are featured on the website that accompanies *Mosby's Canadian Textbook for the Support Worker.* These checklists are designed to help you become skilled at performing procedures that affect the quality of care. Consult with your instructor for correct answers to material presented in this workbook and to the website's procedure checklists. (The website for *Mosby's Canadian Textbook for the Support Worker* can be accessed via http://evolve.elsevier.com/Canada/Sorrentino/SupportWorker)

Support workers are important members of the health care team. Completing the exercises in this workbook will increase your knowledge and skills. Our goal is to prepare you to provide the best possible care and to encourage pride in a job well done.

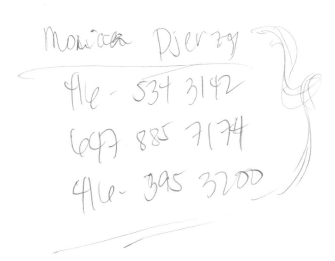

CONTENTS

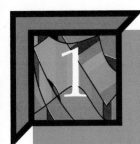

The Role of the Support Worker

True or False

Circle **T** *for true or* **F** *for false. Rewrite all false statements to make them true.*

1. **T** **F**   Most older adults have a serious illness.

   _____

   _____

2. **T** **F**   Most support work with mothers and newborns takes place in the home.

   _____

   _____

3. **T** **F**   Unregulated professions have no official requirements for education.

   _____

   _____

4. **T** **F**   Discretion means keeping private information to yourself.

   _____

   _____

5. **T** **F**   It is okay to discuss your personal problems with a client you have been working with for a long time.

   _____

   _____

6. **T** **F**   Providing compassionate care means treating people with respect.

   _____

   _____

7. **T** **F**   Perfume can cause breathing problems for some clients.

   _____

   _____

8. **T** **F**   Staff members who work together to provide health care for patients are members of the health team.

   _____

   _____

Fill-In-the-Blanks

9. Write the name of the health team member described below in the space provided.

a. _____RN_____ Supervises RPNs and support workers

b. _____Physician_____ Diagnoses and treats diseases and injuries

c. _____Respiratory Therapist_____ Gives respiratory treatments and therapies

d. _____Dietician_____ Assesses and plans for nutritional needs

e. _____PT / physio therapist_____ Assists people with musculoskeletal problems

f. _____Support worker_____ Assists people with learning or retaining skills needed to perform activities of daily living

g. _____Speech Pathologist_____ Treats people with speech, voice, hearing, communication, and swallowing disorders

h. _____Spiritual Advisor_____ Assists people with their spiritual needs

i. _____Social Worker_____ Helps clients and families with social and emotional issues affecting illness and recovery

10. Activities of daily living include

a. _Bathing_

b. _dressing_

c. _eating_

d. _bowel movement_

11. Support workers' responsibilities can be grouped into five categories:

a. _Preserve dignity_

b. _Live independently_

c. _Express their Preference_

d. _preserve privacy_

e. _to be safe from harm_

12. A person receiving care in a hospital is called a

_____patient_____ ;

in a residential facility is called a

_____resident_____ ;

in the community is called a

_____client_____ .

13. The letters in the acronym DIPPS stand for

a. _Dignity_

b. _Independence_

c. _Privacy_

d. _Preference_

e. _Safety_

14. To be a true professional, you should demonstrate

   a. _positive attitude_

   b. _sense of responsibility_

   c. _professional appearance_

   d. _discretion about client information_

   e. _acceptable speech & language_

15. Practices for a professional appearance include

   a. _clothes_

   b. _grooming_

   c. _hygiene_

   d. _____

   e. _____

16. When solving problems, what things should you consider?

   a. _priorities of support work_

   b. _client's viewpoint_

   c. _scope of practice_

   d. _supervisor's viewpoint_

17. Where can you find information about your scope of practice?

   a. _training program_

   b. _employer's policy_

   c. _supervisor_

18. The people you support can be grouped according to their problems, needs, and ages. Some of these groups are

   a. _older people_

   b. _people w/ disabilities_

   c. _people w/ medical problems_

   d. _people having surgery_

   e. _people w/ mental health problems_

   f. _people needing rehabilitation_

   g. _children_

Circle the Correct Answer

19. The support worker can maintain a professional appearance by
    a. wearing fashionable jewellery such as a necklace or bracelet.
    b. having fingernails professionally manicured and polished.
    c. wearing a clean, pressed, and mended uniform each day.
    d. using a lightly scented perfume or aftershave.

Independent Learning Activities

1. Answer these questions about health care facilities in your area.
   - How many hospitals are located in your area? How many beds are available in each one?
   - How many long-term care centres do you have in your area? Do they accept all types of patients (for example, by the level of care needed, the disease category, the method of payment for services)? How many beds does each one have?
   - Find out if you have a mental health care hospital in your area. If there are no mental health hospitals, where do people with mental illness receive care?
   - Do you have home health care agencies or hospices in your area? What are their names? Are they connected to area hospitals or do they operate independently?

2. Whom do you know that works in a health care position? What is the person's position? How many years of schooling did the person need to prepare for this position? What future plans does the person have to continue his/her education?

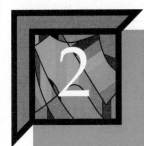

The Canadian Health Care System

Fill-In-the-Blanks

1. The principles of medicare listed in the *Canada Health Act* are

    a. ___Public admin.___

    b. ___Comprehensiveness___

    c. ___Universality___

    d. ___Portability___

    e. ___Accessibility___

2. All home care services provide professional services, which include

    a. ___private home___

    b. ___retirement residence___

    c. ___assisted-living facilities___

    d. _____

3. Health promotion refers to
    ___Strategies that improve___
    ___or maintain health & independence___

4. Disease prevention refers to
    ___Strategies that prevent the___
    ___occurrence of disease & injury___

5. Home care services today provide support to a large range of clients. List some of the clients.

    a. ___Nursing care___

    b. ___Physio therapy___

    c. ___OT___

    d. ___ST___

    e. ___Nutrition counselling___

    f. ___Respiratory therapy___

6. Examples of government policies that promote health and prevent illness are

    a. _____

    b. _____

    c. _____

    d. _____

7. As a support worker, how do you contribute to health promotion?

    _____

    _____

True or False

Circle **T** *for true or* **F** *for false. Rewrite all false statements to make them true.*

8. **T** **F** One of the provincial roles in health care is to deliver health care services to Aboriginal people.

_____

_____

9. **T** **F** The Canadian health care system has seen a shift in focus from home care to hospital care.

_____

_____

10. **T** **F** Patients are being sent home sooner after hospital procedures.

_____

_____

11. **T** **F** Home care enables some people to maintain their health and independence.

_____

_____

12. **T** **F** The federal and provincial governments share health costs.

_____

_____

13. **T** **F** Income and social status does not have an influence on health.

_____

_____

14. **T** **F** People can lose their medicare benefits if they are fired from a job.

_____

15. **T** **F** Support workers provide most support services for home care.

_____

Matching

Match each statement below with the correct year.

16. _1930_ No health insurance in Canada.   1961

17. _1947_ Saskatchewan introduced an insurance plan to cover hospital costs.   1947

18. _1972_ All provinces covered medical services provided outside hospitals.   1930

19. _1961_ All provinces covered in-patient hospital care.   1972

*For the following, mark **P** to indicate professional services or **S** for support services.*

20. __P__   Nursing care

21. __P__   Physiotherapy

22. __S__   Personal care

23. __S__   Social work

24. __S__   Assistance with ADL

25. __P__   Speech therapy

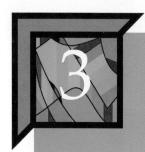

Workplace Settings

Matching

Match the type of service with the correct descriptions.

1. _Palliative care_   Serves people and families living with progressive and life-threatening illness

2. _Long term care_   Provides services to people who do not need hospital care but cannot care for themselves at home

3. _Acute care_   Provides temporary care of a person with a serious illness or disability

4. _Acute care_   Provides services to people with immediate health issues

5. _Respite care_   Serves people with stable conditions who may require complex equipment and care measures

6. _Rehabilitation_   Provides therapies and education designed to restore or improve a person's independence

7. _Mental health services_   Provides services for people with mental disorders

8. _home care_   Provides care to people in their home

a. Respite care

b. Home care

c. Palliative care

d. Acute care

e. Long-term care

f. Subacute care

g. Rehabilitation

h. Mental health services

Fill-In-the-Blanks

9. A chronic illness is _An ongoing illness,_ _slow or gradual in onset, usual_ _there is no known cure. grows_ _worse over time._

   An example of a chronic illness is

   diabete, Multiple Sclerosis,
   Alzheimer's dis.

10. An acute illness is described as
    appear suddenly & lasts
    a short time, symptoms
    can be severe .

    An example of an acute illness is

    Pneumonia & Influenza .

11. Working in home care presents issues and challenges such as

    a. _working on your own_

    b. _may take direction from_ _different health care prof._

    c. _maintaining prof'l boundaries_

    d. _Providing for client &_ _personal safety_

12. What types of services do community day programs offer?

    a. _arts & crafts_

    b. _social visits_

    c. _film, board or card games_

13. A residential facility provides care to

    resident (type of resident)

14. The goals of long-term care are

    _____

    _____

    _____

    _____

True or False

*Circle **T** for true or **F** for false. Rewrite all false statements to make them true.*

15. T **F** Retirement residences are financed by the government.

    In some province, they are

    privately operated

16. **T** F Support workers are responsible for 80% of the total hours worked by all home care workers.

    _____

    _____

17. **T** F Some hospitals are hiring support workers.

    _____

    _____

18. T **F** In a community day program, the support worker works independently.

    _____

    _____

19. **T** F Working in a facility requires you to do many tasks in a short period of time.

    _____

    _____

20. **T** F Lack of privacy can lead to loss of self-esteem.

    _____

    _____

21. T **F** Another term for acute care is convalescent care.

    _____

    _____

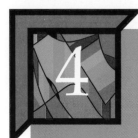

Health, Wellness, Illness, and Disability

Matching

Match the dimension of health with the correct definition.

1. __C__ Is achieved through an active creative mind

2. __a__ Is achieved when the body is strong, fit, and free of disease

3. __b__ Is achieved through stable and satisfactory relationships

4. __e__ Results when people feel good about themselves

5. __d__ Is achieved through the belief in a purpose greater than the self

a. Physical

b. Social

c. Intellectual

d. Spiritual

e. Emotional

Match the illness or disability with the correct definition.

6. __g__ Progressive impairment of all aspects of brain function

7. __c__ A condition affecting joints and/or connective tissue

8. __f__ A disease in which air is trapped inside the lungs

9. __a__ Deterioration of bone tissue

10. __d__ An abnormal growth of cells

11. __e__ Paralysis from the waist down

12. __h__ Body is unable to produce insulin

13. __b__ Paralysis from the neck down

a. Osteoporosis

b. Quadriplegia

c. Arthritis

d. Cancer

e. Paraplegia

f. Emphysema

g. Dementia

h. Diabetes

True or False

Circle **T** *for true or* **F** *for false. Rewrite all false statements to make them true.*

14. **T   F**   A formal group of people who help each other is called a social support system.

_____

_____

15. **T   F**   For some people, spiritual health is closely linked with religion.

_____

_____

16. **T   F**   Shamans are believed to use special powers to aid in the healing process.

_____

_____

17. **T   F**   Illness is the loss of physical or mental function.

_____

_____

18. **T   F**   Self-image is the individual's perception of himself or herself.

_____

_____

19. **T   F**   Discrimination is a characteristic that marks a person as different or flawed.

_____

_____

20. **T   F**   It is less stressful to your client if you make all the decisions.

_____

_____

21. **T   F**   Changes in sexual function greatly affect some people.

_____

_____

Fill-In-the-Blanks

22. Health is defined as a state of

_____.

23. What are the five dimensions of health?

a. _____

b. _____

c. _____

d. _____

e. _____

24. What factors contribute to physical health?

a. _____

b. _____

c. _____

d. _____

e. _____

25. How can you promote intellectual health for your residents?

a. _____

b. _____

c. _____

d. _____

26. What are some of the factors affecting a person's experience of illness or disability?

    a. _____

    b. _____

    c. _____

    d. _____

    e. _____

27. Common reactions to illness or disability are

    a. _____

    b. _____

    c. _____

    d. _____

    e. _____

28. What are some of the changes and losses associated with illness and disability?

    a. _____

    b. _____

    c. _____

    d. _____

    e. _____

    f. _____

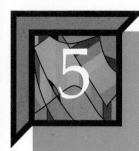

Working with Others

Matching

Match the terms with the correct definition.

1. _e_ To work together toward a common goal   a. Delegation

2. _a_ Transfer of function   b. Case manager

3. _f_ The nurse on duty for that shift   c. Task

4. _b_ Assess client's needs in the community   d. Team leader

5. _d_ Usually an RN in a facility   e. Collaborate

6. _c_ A function you perform for the client   f. Charge nurse

7. _g_ The legal right   g. Authority

Match the correct Right of Delegation for Assistive Personnel with the question the support worker should ask before performing an assigned task.

8. _b_ Do you have the equipment and supplies to complete the task safely?   a. Right task

9. _c_ Are you comfortable performing the task?   b. Right circumstances

10. _e_ Is an RN available if the person's condition changes or if problems occur?   c. Right person

11. _c_ Were you trained to do the task?   d. Right directions or communications

12. _d_ Did you review the task with an RN?

13. _e_ Is an RN available to answer any questions?   e. Right supervision

14. _b_ Do you understand the purposes of the task for the person?

15. _e_ Do you have concerns about performing the task?

16. _d_ Do you understand what the RN expects?

17. _a_ Is the task in your job description?

True or False

Circle **T** *for true or* **F** *for false. Rewrite all false statements to make them true.*

18. **T**   **F**   Only an RN can delegate a task to you.

_____

_____

19. **T**   **F**   RPNs are not allowed to supervise support workers.

_____

_____

20. **T**   **F**   It is okay to discuss work problems with your client as long as you do not use proper names.

_____

_____

21. **T**   **F**   When you agree to perform a task, you are responsible for your own actions.

_____

_____

22. **T**   **F**   You may refuse a delegated task if you do not want to do the task.

_____

_____

23. **T**   **F**   An RN may delegate an RPN to teach you a task.

_____

_____

24. **T**   **F**   Support workers are allowed to perform procedures below the skin surface.

_____

_____

Circle the Correct Answer

25. When the RN delegates a task to a support worker, who is accountable for the delegated task?
    a. The RN
    b. The support worker
    c. The RPN
    d. The doctor

26. Each of the following is one of the five rights of delegation *except*
    a. right directions and communication.
    b. right supervision.
    c. right equipment.
    d. right circumstances.

27. The support worker may refuse to perform a task if he/she
    a. was not prepared to perform the task safely.
    b. does not know the patient or resident.
    c. knows the task will cause him/her to stay past the end of the shift.
    d. does not like the RN who asks him/her to perform the task.

28. Which of the following activities would be acceptable while you are at work?
    a. Making a copy of your cancelled cheque on the photocopier
    b. Planning to eat lunch with your sister
    c. Leaving a half hour early for a doctor's appointment
    d. None of the above

Fill-In-the-Blanks

29. What are some of the benefits of working on a team?

    a. _____

    b. _____

    c. _____

    d. _____

    e. _____

30. Who is usually included on a team in a long-term care facility?

    a. _____

    b. _____

    c. _____

    d. _____

    e. _____

    f. _____

31. When RNs delegate a task to you in a facility, they are required to

    a. _____

    b. _____

    c. _____

32. What are some of the factors affecting delegation decisions?

    a. _____

    b. _____

    c. _____

    d. _____

    e. _____

    f. _____

33. Teams in home care usually include

    a. _____

    b. _____

    c. _____

    d. _____

    e. _____

    f. _____

    g. _____

    h. _____

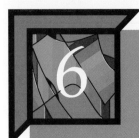

Working with Clients and Their Families

Matching

Match the psychosocial task as described by Erikson's theory with the age range at which it occurs.

1. ___g___ Generativity versus stagnation

2. ___e___ Initiative versus guilt

3. ___d___ Identity versus role confusion

4. ___f___ Integrity versus despair

5. ___h___ Trust versus mistrust

6. ___a___ Competence versus inferiority

7. ___c___ Intimacy versus isolation

8. ___b___ Autonomy versus doubt

a. 6–12 years

b. 1–3 years

c. 20–40 years

d. 12–19 years

e. 3–6 years

f. 65 years on

g. 40–65 years

h. 0–1 year

Match one of Maslow's hierarchy of needs with each of the words or phrases.

9. ___a___ Clothing

10. ___c___ Closeness

11. ___e___ Experiencing one's potential

12. ___a___ Food

13. ___b___ Protection from harm

14. ___c___ Affection

15. ___a___ Water

16. ___c___ Meaningful relationships

17. ___a___ Rest

18. ___a___ Elimination

19. ___d___ Opinion of self

20. ___a___ Shelter

a. Physical

b. Safety

c. Love and belonging

d. Self-esteem

e. Self-actualization

Fill-In-the-Blanks

21. What factors can influence psychosocial health?

     a. _____

     b. _____

     c. _____

     d. _____

22. How can you meet your client's safety needs when doing a procedure?

     a. _____

     b. _____

     c. _____

     d. _____

23. List some of the different types of families you may work with.

     a. _____

     b. _____

     c. _____

     d. _____

     e. _____

24. How can you show your client respect?

     a. _____

     b. _____

     c. _____

     d. _____

25. Describe the difference between a professional helping relationship and a friendship.

     _____

     _____

     _____

Labelling

26. Label each section of the pyramid with the basic need according to Maslow.

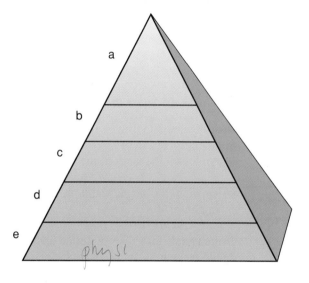

     a. _physical_____

     b. _safety_____

     c. _love & belonging_____

     d. _self esteem_____

     e. _self actualization_____

7

Client Care: Planning, Processes, Reporting, and Recording

Matching

Match the following statements with one of the key terms related to communication.

1. __e__ Identification of a disease or condition by a doctor

2. __f__ Determines if the goals in the care plan have been met

3. __c__ Statement describing a health problem that can be treated by nursing measures

4. __b__ Written guide that gives direction about the care and services a person should receive

5. __d__ Method used by nurses to plan and deliver nursing care

6. __a__ Action taken by a nursing team member to help person reach a goal

a. Nursing care plan

b. Nursing diagnosis

c. Nursing intervention

d. Care planning process

e. Medical diagnosis

f. Evaluation

Circle the Correct Answer

7. Which of these is *not* a rule of communication?
   a. Use words that have only one meaning
   b. Give very detailed and lengthy explanation
   c. Be specific and concise when giving information
   d. Organize information in a logical manner

8. What information is *not* included on the graphic sheet?
   a. Temperature, pulse, respirations
   b. Bowel sounds
   c. Height and weight
   d. Bowel movements

9. The Kardex is a
   a. part of the medical record (chart).
   b. sheet used to record measurements or observations.
   c. written description of nursing care given.
   d. summary of treatments, diagnosis, and routine care measures.

10. Which of these is a question about an activity of daily living?
    a. Can the person perform personal care without help?
    b. How much food on the tray is eaten?
    c. What is the frequency of bowel movements?

18

d. Can the person move arms and legs?

11. A purpose of a team meeting is to
a. identify the medical diagnosis.
b. develop or revise a person's nursing care plan for effective care.
c. share end-of-shift report.
d. chart day-to-day care of the person.

Fill-In-the-Blanks

12. What are the four senses you use to obtain information about a patient?

a. _____
b. _____
c. _____
d. _____

13. When a person reports things you cannot observe by using your senses, they are called symptoms or _____ data.

14. When you can obtain information about a person with your senses, it is called signs or _____ data.

15. The following words or phrases are either subjective or objective data. In the blank next to each one, place an "S" for subjective or an "O" for objective.

a. _____ Sleepy   f. _____ Gas pain
b. _____ Chest pain   g. _____ Pain when urinating
c. _____ Skin cool   h. _____ Productive cough
d. _____ Bruises   i. _____ Breath has fruity odour
e. _____ Difficulty breathing j. _____ Rapid pulse and shallow breathing

16. The following statements are either subjective or objective. Place an "S" for a subjective statement or an "O" for an objective statement.

a. _____ Mr. Jones states he is cold.
b. _____ Mary has red hair.
c. _____ Mrs. Smith says she has pain in her right shoulder.
d. _____ Temperature 37.6° C (99.6° F), pulse 72, respirations 16
e. _____ Mr. Green ate all of his breakfast.
f. _____ Mrs. Foster says she is anxious about having surgery.

17. Next to each of the following, write the time using the 24-hour clock.

a. _____ 11:00 a.m.   g. _____ 3:00 a.m.
b. _____ 8:00 a.m.   h. _____ 4:50 a.m.
c. _____ 4:00 p.m.   i. _____ 5:30 p.m.
d. _____ 7:30 a.m.   j. _____ 10:45 p.m.
e. _____ 6:45 p.m.   k. _____ 11:55 p.m.
f. _____ 12 noon   l. _____ 9:15 p.m.

18. When you write entries in the chart, you sign your name and _____.

19. What basic observations will give you information about a person?

   a. _____

   b. _____

   c. _____

   d. _____

   e. _____

   f. _____

   g. _____

   h. _____

   i. _____

20. What basic observations can you make to determine a person's ability to respond?

   a. _____

   b. _____

   c. _____

   d. _____

   e. _____

   f. _____

   g. _____

   h. _____

21. What observations will help to determine whether a person has normal movement?

   a. _____

   b. _____

   c. _____

   d. _____

22. What words help a person to describe his/her pain?

   a. _____

   b. _____

   c. _____

   d. _____

   e. _____

   f. _____

   g. _____

   h. _____

23. What observations should be made about a person's respirations?

   a. _____

   b. _____

   c. _____

   d. _____

   e. _____

24. When observing the skin, what questions should be asked?

   a. _____

   b. _____

   c. _____

   d. _____

   e. _____

   f. _____

   g. _____

   h. _____

25. What observations are important to determine how the bowels and bladder are functioning?

   a. _____

   b. _____

   c. _____

   d. _____

   e. _____

   f. _____

   g. _____

   h. _____

   i. _____

   j. _____

26. What activities of daily living should be observed?

   a. _____

   b. _____

   c. _____

   d. _____

   e. _____

27. When reporting to the nurse, you should

   a. Be _____, _____,

     and _____.

   b. Tell the nurse the person's _____,

     _____, and _____.

   c. Report only _____.

   d. Give reports as often as _____

     _____.

   e. Immediately report _____

     _____.

   f. Use progress notes to record _____

     _____.

28. Use the chart as a guide and convert the following times. Convert *a* through *d* from conventional time to the 24-hour clock. Convert *e* through *h* from the 24-hour clock to conventional time.

   a. 2:00 a.m.=_____

   b. 10:30 a.m.=_____

   c. 5:00 a.m.=_____

   d. 9:30 a.m.=_____

   e. 0600=_____ **a.m. p.m.**
     (circle one)

   f. 1145=_____ **a.m. p.m.**
     (circle one)

   g. 1800=_____ **a.m. p.m.**
     (circle one)

   h. 2200=_____ **a.m. p.m.**
     (circle one)

True or False

*Circle **T** for true or **F** for false. Rewrite all false statements to make them true. The statements apply to rule for recording.*

29. **T** **F** Write notes in pencil.

   _____

   _____

30. **T** **F** Include the date whenever a recording is made.

   _____

   _____

31. **T** **F** Make sure writing is legible and neat.

_____

_____

32. **T   F**   Use any abbreviations needed to shorten entry.

_____

_____

33. **T   F**   Use correct spelling, grammar, and punctuation.

_____

_____

34. **T   F**   Use eraser or correction fluid if you make an error.

_____

_____

35. **T   F**   Sign all entries with your name and title as required by the agency.

_____

_____

36. **T   F**   Skip lines between entries.

_____

_____

37. **T   F**   Make sure each form is stamped with person's name.

_____

_____

38. **T   F**   Record what you or others did or observed.

_____

_____

39. **T   F**   Chart all care and treatments early in the shift before beginning work.

_____

_____

40. **T   F**   Record your observations, interpretations, and judgments.

_____

_____

41. **T   F**   Record in a logical and sequential manner.

_____

_____

42. **T   F**   Avoid terms with more than one meaning.

_____

_____

43. **T   F**   Paraphrase the person's words to make the meaning more understandable.

_____

_____

44. **T   F**   Chart any changes from normal or changes in the person's condition.

_____

_____

45. **T   F**   Omit unimportant information.

_____

_____

46. **T   F**   Record safety measures used in caring for the person.

_____

_____

Independent Learning Activities

Class Experiment

It is often difficult to describe fluids in a clear and precise manner. Set up the following examples that imitate situations where you need to describe intake, output, or drainage. Describe as accurately as possible what you see in terms of amounts, colours, and textures. Compare your notes with classmates to see if you are using words that all have the same meaning. What words were used that were clear to understand? What words were used that had more than one meaning?

- Bloody drainage: Mix a teaspoon of ketchup and a teaspoon of water. Pour onto the centre of a paper napkin.
- Urine: Pour a tablespoon of tea into the centre of a paper towel.
- Bleeding: Smear a teaspoon of red jelly in the centre of a paper towel.
- Broth: Pour a half cup of tea into a bowl.

Matching

Substance	Observations
Bloody drainage	
Urine	
Bleeding	
Broth	

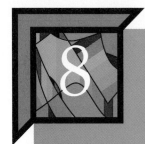

8

Managing Stress, Time, and Problems

Match the term with the definition.

1. _b_   Giving some acceptable reason or excuse for one's behaviour or actions

2. _____   Transferring one's behaviour or emotions from one person, place, or thing to another

         b. Denial

         c. Displacement

3. _____   Expressing or changing an emotion into a physical symptom

         d. Projection

4. _____   Keeping unpleasant or painful thoughts or experiences from the conscious mind

         e. Regression

5. _____   Directing emotions toward another person or thing that seems safe, rather than toward the person or thing that is the source of the emotions

         f. Rationalization

         g. Repression

6. _____   Refusing to face or accept something that is unpleasant

         h. Reaction formation

7. _____   Acting in a way that is opposite to what one truly feels

8. _____   Retreating or moving back to an earlier time or condition

a. Conversion

True or False

*Circle **T** for true or **F** for false. Rewrite all false statements to make them true.*

9. **T**   **F**   Stressors over a short period of time can cause a chronic illness.

    _____

    _____

10. **T**   **F**   You should set weekly goals for yourself.

    _____

    _____

11. **T**   **F**   Getting a promotion can cause stress.

    _____

    _____

12. **T**   **F**   A child usually shows different signs of stress than an adult.

    _____

    _____

13. **T   F**   Time management is essential to reducing stress.

_____

_____

14. **T   F**   There is no point in planning your work a day ahead since things change when you get to work.

_____

_____

15. **T   F**   You don't need to report a conflict with a client if it is resolved.

_____

_____

16. **T   F**   In a home care setting, you must plan your time so you can be on time for the next client.

_____

_____

17. **T   F**   Older adults are less able to cope with stress.

_____

_____

18. **T   F**   All stress is bad for your well-being.

_____

_____

Fill-In-the-Blanks

19. How can you manage stress in your life?

a. _____

b. _____

c. _____

d. _____

20. How can you save time and stay organized?

a. _____

b. _____

c. _____

d. _____

21. What can you do to manage conflict at work?

a. _____

b. _____

c. _____

d. _____

e. _____

f. _____

g. _____

22. Problem solving is a process. Describe this process.

_____

_____

_____

_____

_____

23. What are some common stressors you may face?

    a. _____

    b. _____

    c. _____

    d. _____

    e. _____

24. Physical signs of stress can be

    a. _____

    b. _____

    c. _____

    d. _____

    e. _____

25. Emotional and behavioural signs of stress can include

    a. _____

    b. _____

    c. _____

    d. _____

    e. _____

    f. _____

26. When you realize you have a problem at work, when should you consult your supervisor?

    a. _____

    b. _____

    c. _____

    d. _____

    e. _____

27. When you are setting goals, they must be

    a. _____

    b. _____

    c. _____

    d. _____

    e. _____

28. What steps should be taken to resolve a conflict between two people?

    a. _____

    b. _____

    c. _____

    d. _____

    e. _____

    f. _____

    g. _____

    h. _____

    i. _____

    j. _____

    k. _____

Independent Learning Activities

Set 10 goals for yourself that will help you manage your time and/or stress. Share the goals with someone else. Are your goals specific, measurable, achievable, realistic, and timely?

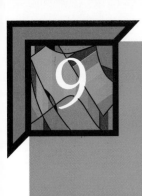

Ethics

Matching

Match the terms with the definition.

1. _e_ Seeking to do no harm
2. _c_ Doing or promoting good
3. _d_ Abuse
4. _b_ All people should be treated in a fair manner
5. _f_ Accidental injury or negligence
6. _a_ Having free choice

a. Autonomy

b. Justice

c. Beneficence

d. Intentional harm

e. Nonmaleficence

f. Unintentional harm

True or False

*Circle **T** for true or **F** for false. Rewrite all false statements to make them true.*

7. **T F** Support workers have a formal code of ethics.

_____

_____

8. **T F** Clients can decide what kind of treatments they want.

_____

_____

9. **T F** You can uphold the principle of justice by being concerned about all clients.

_____

_____

10. **T F** It is okay to talk about a client in the locker room.

_____

_____

11. **T   F**   There is nothing wrong in accepting a dinner invitation from a member of a client's family.

_____

_____

12. **T   F**   A support worker is free to discuss a client's progress or treatment with a close family member.

_____

_____

13. **T   F**   You should not take sides with a client against a family member.

_____

_____

Fill-In-the-Blanks

14. Ethics refers to _moral principles &_
    values that guide us when
    deciding.

15. A sample code of ethics for support workers could include

    a. _____

    b. _____

    c. _____

    d. _____

    e. _____

16. The four basic principles of heath care ethics are

    a. _____

    b. _____

    c. _____

    d._____

17. When confronted with an ethical dilemma, how do you decide what is the right thing to do?

_____

_____

_____

_____

_____

_____

18. What do you do if your client's choice may put him/her at risk for injury?

_____

_____

_____

_____

_____

_____

Circle the Correct Answer

19. Ethics is
    a. concerned with what is right and wrong behaviour.
    b. making bad judgments before knowing the facts.
    c. deciding whether a situation is right or wrong based on your own life experiences.
    d. a law telling you what you can and can't do.

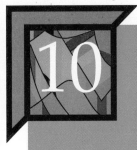

Legislation: The Client's Rights and Your Rights

Matching

Match the words and definitions.

1. _____ What you should or should not do   a. Right

2. _____ Having free choice   b. Legislation

3. _____ Legally responsible   c. Liable

4. _____ Wrongful act committed against another person or the person's property   d. Negligence

5. _____ A body of laws   e. Ethics

6. _____ Failing to act in a competent manner   f. Act

7. _____ Touching a person's body without consent   g. Autonomy

8. _____ Injuring the reputation of a person by making false statements   h. Battery

9. _____ Specific law   i. Defamation

10. _____ Something to which a person is justly entitled   j. Tort

True or False

*Circle **T** for true or **F** for false. Rewrite all false statements to make them true.*

11. **T F** Employment standards and legislation protects you from harassment.

_____

_____

12. **T F** Libel is making false statements in print.

_____

_____

13. **T** **F** The unnecessary use of restraints is false imprisonment.

_____

_____

14. **T** **F** Civil laws deal with relationships between people.

_____

_____

15. **T** **F** A physician can ask you to obtain a consent from a client.

_____

_____

16. **T** **F** You may refuse to do something beyond your scope of practice.

_____

_____

17. **T** **F** A common act of courtesy is one way to respect a client's dignity.

_____

_____

18. **T** **F** It is okay to open a client's mail in case it contains upsetting news.

_____

_____

19. **T** **F** Respecting a person's dignity can encourage independence.

_____

_____

20. **T** **F** It is important to tell the nurse when you leave and return to the unit for meals and breaks.

_____

_____

Circle the Correct Answer

21. If a person has different values or standards than yours, you should
    a. respect each person as an individual.
    b. refuse to care for the person.
    c. try to convince the person that he/she is wrong.
    d. discuss the person's beliefs with others at work or at home.

22. If you are asked to obtain a person's signature on an informed consent, you should
    a. make sure the person is mentally competent.
    b. refuse because this is not a support worker's responsibility.
    c. ask a family member to witness the signature.
    d. call the doctor to witness the signature.

23. If a resident refuses treatment, what action should be taken by the health care facility?
    a. Give the treatment as ordered.
    b. Honour the request and discontinue the treatment.
    c. Find out what the person is refusing and why.
    d. Tell the family that the person must be removed from the facility.

24. A resident tells you he is upset because he believes his treatment was done incorrectly yesterday. Your action is based on which of the following?
    a. He has a right to voice his concerns and have the facility try to correct the matter.
    b. You know the treatment was done correctly.
    c. He complains constantly, so everyone ignores his concerns and questions.
    d. He is confused and forgets what was done yesterday.

25. What rights do residents have?
    a. They may discuss concerns and offer ideas.
    b. They may take part in social, cultural, religious, and community activities.
    c. They may receive support and reassurance from family members and friends.
    d. All of the above.

26. What action by the support worker protects the resident's right to personal possessions?
    a. Throwing away old cards, letters, and magazines to tidy unit
    b. Rearranging personal items so they are more decorative
    c. Getting the resident's permission to look for an item in the closet
    d. Taking a piece of candy from the resident's candy dish when he/she is not present

Fill-In-the-Blanks

27. Basic human rights in Canada include

    a. _____
    b. _____
    c. _____
    d. _____
    e. _____
    f. _____
    g. _____

28. Most long-term care facilities have policies that recognize that residents have the following rights:

    a. _____
    b. _____
    c. _____
    d. _____
    e. _____
    f. _____
    g. _____

29. How can you show respect to your clients?

    a. _____
    b. _____
    c. _____
    d. _____
    e. _____

30. Informed consent is based on _____

    and

    _____.

31. Informed consent should include

    a. _____
    b. _____
    c. _____
    d. _____
    e. _____
    f. _____
    g. _____
    h. _____

32. If a patient complains of chest pain and you do not report this to your supervisor, this is a

    _____ act.

33. Discussing a person's treatment with your best friend invades the person's

    _____

34. List the ways you can protect a client's right to privacy.

    a. _____
    b. _____
    c. _____
    d. _____
    e. _____
    f. _____
    g. _____
    h. _____

35. What can cause negligence?

    a. _____
    b. _____
    c. _____

36. Your best protection against charges of negligence

    is

    _____ .

37. What are some of the laws that protect workers?

    a. _____

    b. _____

    c. _____

    d. _____

    e. _____

    f. _____

38. Who is responsible for job safety?

    _____

    _____

39. What must be done to protect the resident's right to privacy and confidentiality?

    a. The resident's body must not be

       _____

    b. Consent is needed for

       _____ to ob-

       serve.

    c. The resident is allowed to visit

       _____

    d. The resident has the right to

       _____

       and

       _____

       mail without interference.

    e. Information about the resident's

       _____,

       _____,

       and _____ is kept confi-

       dential.

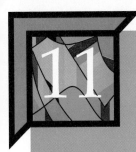

Caring about Culture

Matching

Match the terms and definitions.

1. _____ Characteristics of a group of people

2. _____ An overly simple or exaggerated impression of a person

3. _____ Behaviour that treats people unfairly based on their group membership

4 _____ The area immediately around one's body

5. _____ Groups of people who share similar physical features

6. _____ Groups of people who share a common history

7. _____ An attitude that judges a person based on his/her membership in a group

a. Race

b. Prejudice

c. Ethnic group

d. Culture

e. Personal space

f. Stereotype

g. Discrimination

True or False

*Circle **T** for true or **F** for false. Rewrite all false statements to make them true.*

8. **T   F**   All cultures are comfortable with physical touch.

_____

_____

9. **T   F**   In Western cultures, personal space is about 120 cm (4 feet).

_____

_____

10. **T   F**   Silence can show a sign of respect in some cultures.

_____

_____

11. **T   F**   Some children rebel against the culture of their parents.

_____

_____

12. **T   F**   You should never try to convert your clients to your own belief systems.

_____

_____

13. **T   F**   All folk remedies are harmless.

_____

_____

14. **T   F**   Discrimination leads to prejudice.

_____

_____

15. **T   F**   In Vietnam, men do not shake women's hands.

_____

_____

16. **T   F**   In Asian cultures, eye contact is considered disrespectful.

_____

_____

17. **T   F**   Asking about your client's beliefs and values will help him/her feel valued and respected.

_____

_____

Fill-In-the-Blanks

18. Culture affects a person's beliefs and behaviour toward

    a. _____

    b. _____

    c. _____

    d. _____

19. Nonverbal cues can include

    a. _____

    b. _____

    c. _____

    d. _____

20. Many facial expressions are universal; some of them are

    a. _____

    b. _____

    c. _____

    d. _____

21. An extended family may include

    _____

    _____

    _____

22. How can cultural conflict affect an older person?

    _____

    _____

    _____

23. Religions may promote beliefs and practices related to

    a. _____

    b. _____

    c. _____

    d. _____

    e. _____

    f. _____

    g. _____

24. To be tolerant and understanding of others, you need to understand

    a. _____

    b. _____

    c. _____

25. Asians may conceal negative emotions with a _____.

26. When you communicate with foreign-speaking people, you should

    a. _____

    b. _____

    c. _____

    d. _____

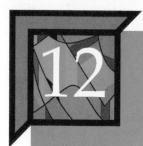

Interpersonal Communications

Matching

Match the description with the correct term.

1. _____ Restating someone's message in your own words

2. _____ Communicating positively and directly without offending others

3. _____ Questions that invite a person to share thoughts

4. _____ Paying close attention to a person's verbal and nonverbal communication

5. _____ Questions that focus on specific information

6. _____ Being attentive to a person's feelings

7. _____ Messages sent without words

8. _____ Limiting the conversation to a certain topic

9. _____ Gestures that send messages to others

10. _____ Spoken word

11. _____ Exchange of information between two people

a. Open-ended questions

b. Nonverbal communication

c. Paraphrasing

d. Verbal communication

e. Closed questions

f. Interpersonal communication

g. Empathetic listening

h. Body language

i. Active listening

j. Focusing

k. Assertiveness

True or False

Circle **T** *for true or* **F** *for false. Rewrite all false statements to make them true.*

12. **T F** The same word can mean something different to two people.

_____

_____

13. **T F** Touch is not a type of communication.

_____

_____

14. **T F** When paraphrasing, expand on the message and use more words to ensure you understand.

_____

_____

15. **T F** Nonverbal clues often reflect a person's true feelings.

_____

_____

16. **T F** Most old people are not aware of your body language.

_____

_____

17. **T F** Closed questions can be answered "yes" or "no."

_____

_____

18. **T F** Focusing is useful when a client rambles.

_____

_____

19. **T F** Short sentences are more clearly understood.

_____

_____

20. **T F** It is not important to be on eye level when communicating.

_____

_____

21. **T F** Using pet names such as "dear" improves communication.

_____

_____

22. **T F** Assertive communication is the same as aggressive communication.

_____

_____

Fill-In-the-Blanks

23. To effectively communicate with words, you need to

a. _____

b. _____

c. _____

d. _____

e. _____

f. _____

g. _____

h. _____

24. Body language includes

    a. _____

    b. _____

    c. _____

    d. _____

    e. _____

25. The communication process involves

    a. _____

    b. _____

    c. _____

    d. _____

26. Guidelines for active listening include

    a. _____

    b. _____

    c. _____

    d. _____

27. You can use open-ended questions to

    a. _____

    b. _____

28. What are some of the barriers to good communications?

    a. _____

    b. _____

    c. _____

    d. _____

    e. _____

    f. _____

    g. _____

29. Certain behaviours can create barriers as well. Some of these are

    a. _____

    b. _____

    c. _____

    d. _____

    e. _____

30. Nonverbal signs of anger include

    a. _____

    b. _____

    c. _____

    d. _____

31. Clients feel safer and more secure during a procedure if you

    a. _____

    b. _____

    c. _____

    d. _____

32. When teaching someone a task, this four-step teaching method works for many people. Describe the steps.

    a. _____

    b. _____

    c. _____

    d. _____

33. What are some of the other guidelines you can use when you are teaching tasks to clients?

    a. _____

    b. _____

    c. _____

    d. _____

    e. _____

34. Gestures, facial expressions, posture, body movements, touch, and appearance are ways of

    _____

    without words.

35. When you hold a person's hand or touch the shoulder to convey caring or warmth, you are using

    _____

    communication.

36. A person who denies having pain but protects a body part by lying in a certain way is using

    _____

    language to communicate.

37. When a support worker frowns or wrinkles his/her nose because the client has body odour, the

    _____

    sends a message through body language.

38. If a support worker tells a person "Don't worry" or "Everything will be okay," this may be a

    _____ to

    effective communication.

39. What are the guidelines for dealing with an angry person?

    a. _____

    b. _____

    c. _____

    d. _____

    e. _____

    f. _____

    g. _____

    h. _____

    i. _____

    j. _____

    k. _____

Body Structure and Function

Matching

Match the following statements with the correct term.

1. _____ Blood vessel that carries blood away from the heart

2. _____ Blood vessel that carries blood back to the heart

3. _____ Tiny blood vessel that allows food, oxygen, and other substances to pass to the cells

4. _____ Basic unit of body structure

5. _____ Group of cells with the same function

6. _____ Group of tissues with the same function

7. _____ Organs that work together to perform special functions

8. _____ Process of physically and chemically breaking down food so it can be absorbed for use by the cells of the body

9. _____ Muscle contractions in the digestive system that move food through the alimentary canal

10. _____ Burning of food for heat and energy by the cells

a. Artery

b. Capillary

c. Cell

d. Digestion

e. Metabolism

f. Organ

g. Peristalsis

h. System

i. Tissue

j. Vein

*Place an **S** in front of the statements that describe a function of the skin. Place an **M** in front of the statements that describe a function of the musculoskeletal system.*

11. _____ Provides a framework

12. _____ Provides a protective covering

13. _____ Regulates body temperature

14. _____ Allows the body to move

15. _____ Gives the body shape

16. _____ Has nerve endings that allow the body to sense pleasant and unpleasant stimulation

Match the following statements with one of the terms related to the digestive and urinary systems.

17. _____ Structure that adds digestive juices to chyme   a. Bladder

18. _____ Semiliquid food mixture formed in stomach   b. Chyme

19. _____ Portion of GI tract that absorbs food   c. Colon

20. _____ Portion of GI tract that absorbs water   d. Duodenum

21. _____ Produces digestive juices   e. Jejunum

22. _____ Produces bile   f. Kidney

23. _____ Basic working unit of the kidney   g. Liver

24. _____ Hollow muscular sac that stores urine   h. Meatus

25. _____ Structure that allows urine to pass from the bladder   i. Nephrons

26. _____ Opening from the bladder at the end of the urethra   j. Pancreas

27. _____ Bean-shaped structure that produces urine   k. Saliva

28. _____ Moistens food particles in the mouth   l. Urethra

Match the action of the hormone with the correct hormone.

29. _____ Released by pancreas and regulates sugar in blood   a. Epinephrine

30. _____ Sex hormone secreted by testes   b. Estrogen

31. _____ Sex hormone secreted by ovaries   c. Insulin

32. _____ Regulates metabolism   d. Parathormone

33. _____ Regulates calcium levels in body   e. Testosterone

34. _____ Stimulates body to produce energy during emergencies   f. Thyroxine

Fill-In-the-Blanks

35. What are the basic structures of the cell?

    a. _____

    b. _____

    c. _____

36. The process of cell division is called _____

    _____ .

37. What are four basic types of tissue and their
    functions?

    a. _____

    _____

    b. _____

    _____

    c. _____

    _____

    d. _____

    _____

38. What does each type of bone do?

    a. Long bones _____

    _____

    b. Short bones _____

    _____

    c. Flat bones _____

    _____

    d. Irregular bones _____

    _____

39. What movements does each joint make?

    a. Ball and socket _____

_____

    b. Hinge _____

    _____

    c. Pivot _____

    _____

40. Skeletal muscles are attached to _____

    _____

    and cause

    _____ of

    body parts.

41. What is the function of the nervous system?

    _____

    _____

42. The pathways that conduct messages to and from

    the brain are contained in the _____

    _____ .

43. What are the five senses?

    a. _____

    b. _____

    c. _____

    d. _____

    e. _____

44. Three small bones in the middle ear _____

    the sound and transmit it to the _____

    _____ . The small bones in

    the middle ear are called the _____ ,

    _____ , and

    _____ .

45. What are the structures that make up the circulatory system?

    a. _____

    b. _____

    c. _____

46. What is the function of the lungs?

    _____

    _____

47. Describe the function of the digestive system.

    _____

    _____

48. The undigested portion of food that passes from the body through the rectum and anus is called _____.

49. Urine is made up of waste products filtered out of the _____.

50. What are the functions of the ovaries?

    a. _____

    b. _____

51. The master gland of the endocrine system is the _____ gland.

52. What effect do these pituitary hormones have on the body?

    a. Growth hormone _____

    b. Thyroid-stimulating hormone (TSH) _____

    c. Adrenocorticotropic hormone (ACTH) _____

    d. Antidiuretic hormone (ADH) _____

    e. Oxytocin _____

53. The major function of the thyroid gland is to regulate _____.

54. The parathyroid glands are important because they regulate the use of _____ by the body.

55. What effect do these adrenal hormones have on the body?

    a. Glucocorticoids _____

    b. Mineralocorticoids _____

56. Explain how special cells and substances in the immune system protect the body.

    a. Antibodies _____

    b. Antigens _____

c. Phagocytes _____

_____

d. Lymphocytes _____

_____

e. B lymphocytes (B cells) _____

_____

f. T lymphocytes (T cells) _____

_____

57. Identify the type of joint in each drawing. Name a joint in the body that moves like each one.

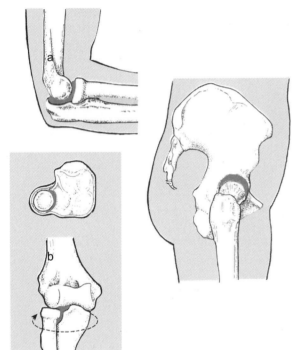

a. _____

b. _____

c. _____

58. Label the parts of the brain indicated on the drawing.

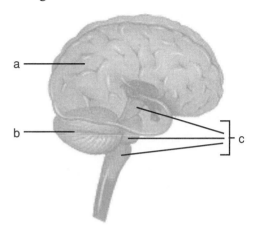

a. _____

b. _____

c. _____

Answer questions 59 and 60 using the following illustration.

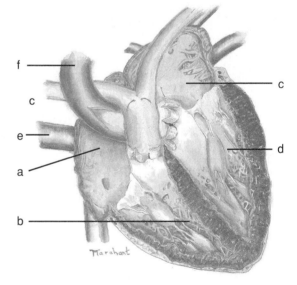

59. Name the structure and function of the six main parts of the heart indicated on the drawing.

a. _____

_____

b. _____

_____

c. _____

_____

d. _____

_____

e. _____

_____

f. _____

_____

60. Use a red pencil or pen and draw arrows to show the pathway of the blood through the heart.

61. Name the structures of the respiratory system indicated on the drawing.

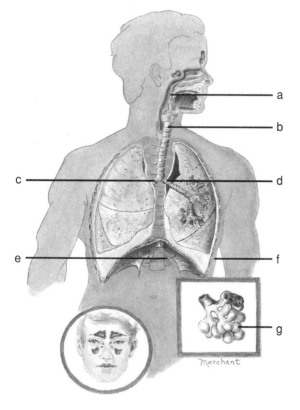

a. _____

b. _____

c. _____

d. _____

e. _____

f. _____

g. _____

62. Name the structures of the digestive system indicated on the drawing.

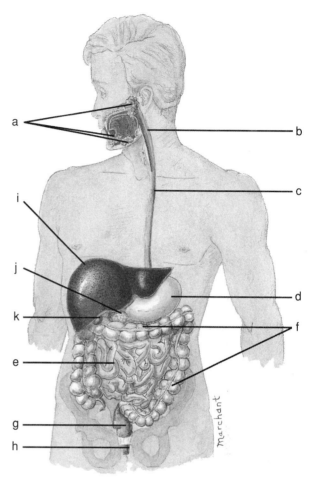

a. _____

b. _____

c. _____

d. _____

e. _____

f. _____

g. _____

h. _____

i. _____

j. _____

k. _____

63. Name the structures of the urinary system indicated on the drawing.

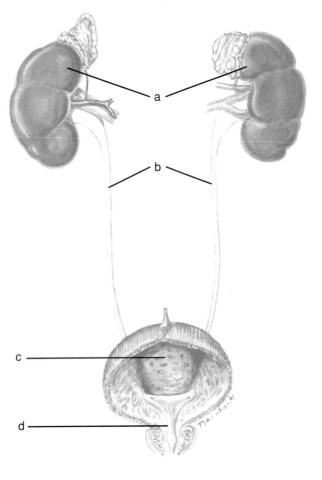

a. _____

b. _____

c. _____

d. _____

64. Name the structures and the functions of the parts of the male reproductive system indicated on the drawing.

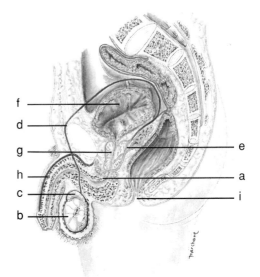

a. _____

_____

b. _____

_____

c. _____

_____

d. _____

_____

e. _____

_____

f. _____

_____

g. _____

_____

h. _____

_____

i. _____

_____

65. Name the structures of the external female genitalia indicated on the drawing.

a. _____

b. _____

c. _____

d. _____

e. _____

f. _____

g. _____

Independent Learning Activities

1. Use your own body and move joints of each type to see how they move.
   - What joint did you use for a ball and socket?
   - What joint moved like a hinge?
   - Which joint did you move in a pivot motion?

2. Listen to your heartbeat using a stethoscope. Find a pulse in your wrist to feel the blood being pumped through an artery.

3. Listen to a friend's chest with a stethoscope. What sound do you hear? What is making that sound?

4. Have you ever heard your stomach "growl" or heard gurgling noises in your abdomen when you were sitting quietly? What makes that sound? What is the medical term for this action? Listen to your lower abdomen with a stethoscope to hear the sounds.

5. Look at a friend's eye in a dimly lit room and observe the size of the pupils. Now shine a light in the eye. What happens to the pupil? What happens when you move the light away from the eye?

NOTE: Students are responsible only for those terms mentioned in the text. Additional terms used in labelling figures throughout this chapter are for illustrative purposes only.

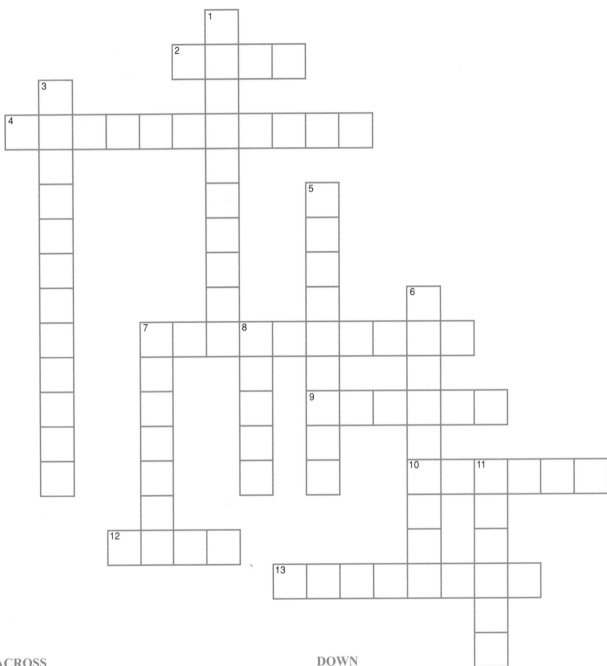

ACROSS

2. Blood vessel that carries blood back to the heart
4. Involuntary muscle contractions in the digestive system that move food through the alimentary canal
7. Substance in red blood cells that carries oxygen and gives blood its colour
9. Blood vessel that carries blood away from heart
10. Group of cells with the same function
12. Basic unit of body structure
13. Protection against a disease or infection; the person will not get or be affected by the disease

DOWN

1. Burning of food for heat and energy by the cells
3. Process in which the lining of the uterus breaks up and is discharged from the body through the vagina
5. Tiny blood vessel; food, oxygen, and other substances pass from the capillaries to the cells
6. Process of physically and chemically breaking down food so that it can be absorbed for use by the cells
7. Chemical substance secreted by the glands into the bloodstream
8. Group of tissues with the same function
11. Organs that work together to perform special functions

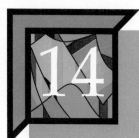

Growth and Development

Fill-In-the-Blanks

According to your textbook, at what age is a child expected to develop each of the following skills?

1. _____ Speaks in short sentences

2. _____ Usually protective of younger brothers and sisters

3. _____ Child learns to write rather than print

4. _____ Smiles and follows objects with the eyes

5. _____ Can eat table food

6. _____ Capable of bladder control during the day

7. _____ Can hold a rattle

8. _____ Knows male and female bodies are different

9. _____ Reacts to the word "no"

10. _____ Begins to bite and chew finger foods

11. _____ Plays with the toes

12. What are the six basic principles of growth and development?

    a. _____

    _____

    b. _____

    _____

c. _____

_____

d. _____

_____

e. _____

_____

f. _____

_____

13. Physical changes that can be measured and occur in a steady and organized manner are called

    _____.

14. A change in psychological and social functioning is called _____.

15. A _____ is a baby in the first 4 weeks after birth.

16. The 4-year-old child has a strong preference for the parent of the _____ sex.

17. At what age are peer-group activities and opinions important to the child?

    _____

18. Adolescence begins when reproductive organs begin to function. What is this event called?

_____

19. During _____,
hobbies and pastimes can be pursued as more free time is available.

20. What stage of growth and development includes the following developmental tasks?

_____

- Adjusting to physical changes
- Having grown children
- Developing leisure-time activities
- Relating to aging parents

21. What stage of growth and development includes the following developmental tasks?

_____

- Increasing the ability to communicate and understand others
- Performing self-care activities
- Learning the differences between the sexes and developing sexual modesty
- Learning right from wrong and good from bad
- Learning to play with others
- Developing family relationships

Identify the age when each behaviour or physical change usually occurs.

22. _____ Do not like being teased or criticized and are sensitive about how others treat them

23. _____ Temper tantrums and saying "no" are common

24. _____ In girls, pelvis becomes broader, fat appears on hips and chest, and budding of breasts occurs

25. _____ Movements are uncoordinated and lack purpose

26. _____ Select partner and learn to live together, develop intimate relationships

27. _____ May be able to stand when holding onto something

28. _____ Menarche occurs, breasts increase in size, hair appears in pubic and axillary areas

29. _____ Bowel training usually is complete

30. _____ Awkward movements occur because of rapid growth in height and weight

31. _____ Recognizes that male and female bodies are different

32. _____ More permanent teeth appear; movements are faster and more graceful

33. _____ Weight control becomes a problem as metabolism and physical activity slow down

34. _____ May cheat to win, but they like rules and try to follow them

35. _____ Responsible for aging parents and deals with death of parents

36. _____ Makes decision to have children and plans number of children

37. _____ Baby teeth are lost, and replacement with permanent teeth begins

Matching

Match the following statements with the correct reflex of an infant. You can use a reflex more than once to answer.

38. _____ Produced by touching the cheeks		a. Moro (startle) reflex
39. _____ When cheek is touched, baby turns head in the direction of touch		b. Rooting reflex
40. _____ A loud noise causes infant to throw arms apart and extend legs		c. Sucking reflex
41. _____ When palm of hand is touched, baby closes fingers around object		d. Grasping reflex
42. _____ Guides baby's mouth to nipple		
43. _____ Disappears by the third month		

Match the developmental task with the correct age group. You can use an age group more than once to answer.

44. _____ Accepting the changes in body and appearance

45. _____ Developing leisure-time activities

46. _____ Gaining control of bowel and bladder functions

47. _____ Becoming independent from parents and adults

48. _____ Learning to eat solid foods

49. _____ Developing new friends and relationships

50. _____ Learning how to study

51. _____ Learning to get along with peers

52. _____ Increasing ability to communicate and understand others

53. _____ Tolerating separation from primary caregiver

54. _____ Learning to live with a partner

55. _____ Developing moral and ethical behaviour

56. _____ Learning basic reading, writing, and arithmetic skills

57. _____ Developing stable sleep and feeding patterns

58. _____ Performing self-care activities

59. _____ Using words to communicate with others

60. _____ Relating to aging parents

61. _____ Accepting male or female role appropriate for one's age

62. _____ Beginning to have emotional relationships with primary caregivers, brothers, and sisters

a. Infancy (birth to 1 year)

b. Toddler (1 to 3 years)

c. Preschooler (3 to 6 years)

d. Middle childhood (6 to 8 years)

e. Late childhood (9 to 12 years)

f. Adolescence (12 to 18 years)

g. Young adulthood (18 to 40 years)

h. Middle adulthood (40 to 65 years)

i. Late adulthood (65 years and older)

Independent Learning Activities

1. Observe or interview one person in three or four of the age groups discussed in the textbook. (For example, you may want to observe three or four children of different age groups, or two children and two adults in different age groups.) Find out how the person has met or is working toward meeting the developmental tasks for each group.

2. Choose an age group between infancy and adolescence. Observe two or more children in the group. Compare how children of about the same age are meeting the developmental tasks. What differences or similarities are observed?

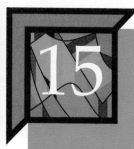

Caring for Older Adults

Matching

Match the examples given with the benefits of working or retiring and the negative aspects of retirement.

1. _____ Time to travel

2. _____ More leisure time

3. _____ Poor health and aging

4. _____ Increased medical bills with less income

5. _____ Personal fulfillment and usefulness

6. _____ Friendship formed with co-workers

7. _____ Reduced income forces lifestyle changes

8. _____ Time to do as you wish

9. _____ Meets basic needs of love and belonging and self-esteem

10. _____ Reward for lifetime of work

a. Benefit of retirement

b. Negative aspect of retirement

c. Benefit of working

Match the effects of aging with the correct type of change. Some may have more than one answer.

11. _____ Greying hair

12. _____ Preparing for one's own death

13. _____ Death of a partner

14. _____ Slower movements

15. _____ Retirement

a. Physical

b. Psychological

c. Social

Match the statement about physical changes in the older person with the body system affected.

16. _____   Decrease in bone strength

17. _____   Change in sleeping patterns

18. _____   Less blood flows through narrowed arteries

19. _____   Folds, lines, and wrinkles appear

20. _____   Lung tissue becomes less elastic

21. _____   Decreased appetite

22. _____   Urine becomes concentrated

23. _____   Increased sensitivity to cold

24. _____   Reduced sense of touch

a. Integumentary

b. Musculoskeletal

c. Nervous

d. Cardiovascular

e. Respiratory

f. Digestive

g. Urinary

True or False

Circle T *if the statement promotes a person's sexuality and* F *if it does not. Rewrite all false statements to make them true.*

25. **T   F**   Encourage the person to wear a hospital gown at all times.

_____

_____

26. **T   F**   Protect the person's right to privacy.

_____

_____

27. **T   F**   Encourage the person to get counselling if the person's sexual attitudes are different from yours.

_____

_____

28. **T   F**   Knock before you enter a room.

_____

_____

29. **T   F**   Allow older people the right to be sexual.

_____

_____

30. **T   F**   Discourage single older people from developing new relationships.

_____

_____

31. **T   F**   Allow couples in the long-term care facility to share the same room.

_____

_____

32. **T   F**   Discourage a woman from shaving her underarms and legs.

_____

_____

Circle the Correct Answer

33. Which of these statements does *not* describe sexuality?
    a. It involves the whole personality and the body
    b. It is influenced by social, cultural, and spiritual factors
    c. It is present from birth
    d. It is done for pleasure or to produce children

34. Which of these statements is *true* about sexuality and the older person?
    a. After menopause, women are no longer interested in having sexual relations
    b. A man cannot have an erection as he gets older
    c. Sexual relationships are psychologically and physically important to the older person
    d. Orgasm may be less intense and longer in duration

Fill-In-the-Blanks

35. The young-old are between the ages of

    _____ and _____ .

36. The middle-old are between the ages of

    _____ and _____ .

37. The _____

    are people over the age of 85.

38. What are two common causes of loneliness in the older person?

    a. _____

    b. _____

39. What happens to the roles of children and parents as the parent ages?

    _____

40. What are some ways loneliness in older people can be prevented?

    a. _____

    b. _____

    c. _____

41. Why are there usually more widows than widowers?

    _____

42. When a partner dies, how is the other partner affected?

    a. Serious _____ and

       _____ problems may occur.

    b. May lose _____

       or attempt _____ .

43. Why do older people who speak a foreign language often have greater loneliness and isolation than others?

    a. Relatives and friends who share cultural values

       may _____ .

    b. Person may not have anyone _____

       _____ and may

       not _____ .

44. How do these physical changes affect the safety of the older person?

    a. Skin is fragile and easily injured _____

       _____ .

    b. Fewer nerve endings _____

       _____ .

    c. Decreasing strength and muscle atrophy

       _____ .

    d. Bones become brittle _____

       _____ .

    e. Reduced sense of touch and pain _____

       _____ .

    f. Reduced blood flow to brain, loss of brain cells

       _____ .

45. Older people often complain of feeling cold. What are some ways you can safely provide warmth?

    a. _____

    b. _____

    c. _____

46. How can loss of bone and muscle strength be slowed?

    a. _____

    b. _____

47. Touch and sensitivity to _____

    and _____

    are reduced with aging.

48. What body system will be affected by the care measures described?

    a. Performing range-of-motion exercises _____

    _____.

    b. Providing a sweater and a lap blanket for a

    person who is cold _____

    _____

    c. Allowing the older person to rest or nap more

    during the day _____

    _____

    d. Placing the person in a semi-Fowler's position

    _____

49. The older person needs foods that prevent

    _____ and

    _____ changes.

50. Urine may be more concentrated because of

    _____ and

    _____.

51. Urinary frequency or urgency may occur because

    _____ weakens

    and _____ decreases.

52. Men may have _____

    or _____

    because of prostate gland enlargement.

53. The support worker can help the person at risk for

    urinary tract infections by providing _____

    _____.

54. Why should you make sure an older person reduces fluid intake after 5:00 p.m.?

    _____

55. How can the support worker promote normal breathing in the older person?

    a. _____

    b. _____

    c. _____

56. What are some ways that an older person may express closeness and intimacy without having intercourse?

    a. _____

    b. _____

    c. _____

    d. _____

Circle the Correct Answer

57. Which of the following physical changes is most likely to cause confusion or behavioural changes in an older person?
    a. Respiratory infections
    b. Lack of exercise
    c. Blood flow to brain is reduced
    d. Poor fluid intake

58. Why does an older person usually require a bath only twice a week?
    a. Less exercise is done so frequent bathing is unnecessary
    b. Fewer baths decrease the possibility of injury from falls in the tub
    c. Skin becomes drier with aging and is easily damaged by frequent bathing
    d. Muscles atrophy and strength is reduced

59. Why should you avoid applying heat to the feet of an older person?
    a. The skin is dry and has decreased oil glands
    b. More fold lines and wrinkles appear in the skin
    c. The feet may become infected more easily
    d. Decreased sensitivity to heat may increase risk of burns

60. Older people often complain that food has no taste. This happens because
    a. memory is shorter in older people.
    b. the number of taste buds decrease with aging.
    c. the ability to feel heat and cold decreases.
    d. a progressive loss of brain cells occurs.

Independent Learning Activities

1. Interview an older person who lives independently. What concerns does the person have about remaining independent? Use these suggestions to guide your conversation.
   - What physical problems does the person have, if any?
   - What ways does the person use to provide safety?
   - What comfort measures are used to decrease pain or help the person sleep?
   - How does the person get to the store for groceries or other needs?
   - How are needs for socialization met?

2. Interview an older person and talk about life when he/she was young. Observe facial expressions and tone of voice when the person talks about events remembered. What changes do you see from the usual appearance of the person? Compare how well the person remembers events of long ago with events that occurred recently. How do you feel about the person after hearing about the person's youth? Use these suggestions to guide your conversation.
   - What did the person do for a living?
   - Ask to see any pictures of the person from long ago.
   - What stories about family and friends make the person happy? Sad?
   - Ask about historical events the person remembers.

16

Safety

Matching

Match the safety measure used with the correct risk factor.

1. __d__ Teach children not to eat plants, unknown foods, leaves, stems, seeds, berries, nuts, or bark

2. __a__ Measure the temperature of bath water

3. __c__ Keep person's room free of clutter

4. __c__ Keep one hand on child lying on table if you must look away

5. __a__ Do not allow smoking in bed

6. __b__ Do not prop baby bottle with rolled up towel or blanket

7. __b__ Never leave children unattended in bathtub

8. __c__ Use nonslip strips on the floor next to the bed and in bathroom

9. __a__ Open doors and windows if you notice gas odours

10. __d__ Store cleaners, medicines, and hazardous substances in original containers

11. __a__ Turn pot and pan handles so they point inward from front of stove

12. __b__ Keep cords for drapes, blinds, and shades out of reach of children

a. Burns

b. Suffocation

c. Falls

d. Poisoning

Match the accident risk factor with the example or reason accidents can occur because of the risk factor.

13. _____ Can harm themselves or others because they cannot understand what is happening

14. ___b___ May take wrong medication or dosage, or poison self because the person cannot read labels

15. ___d___ Having problem smelling smoke or gas

16. ___c___ Cannot hear fire alarms or sirens, so cannot move to safety

17. ___g___ Helpless, have not learned difference between safety and danger

18. ___e___ Cannot react or respond to people, place, or things

19. ___e___ May be aware of danger, but unable to move to safety

20. ___g___ Movements slower and less steady, balance affected

21. ___b___ Can trip on toys, rugs, furniture, electric cords

22. ___d___ Easily burned because of problems sensing heat and cold

23. ___c___ May take wrong medication or dosage because cannot hear explanations or instructions

24. ___d___ Cannot sense heat, cold, or pain

25. ___g___ Side effects can cause loss of balance, confusion, or loss of coordination

a. Aware of surroundings

b. Vision

c. Hearing

d. Smell or touch

e. Paralysis

f. Medications

g. Age

Fill-In-the-Blanks

26. How can you help to prevent injuries in infants and children when using the following items?

    a. Baby walker _____

    _____

    b. High chair _____

    _____

    c. Cribs _____

    _____

    d. Electric appliances, equipment _____

    _____

    e. Strings, cords _____

    _____

    f. Medications, cleaners _____

    _____

    g. Clothing _____

    _____

27. List ways to prevent children from drowning in or around the home. (Do not include pools, spas, whirlpools, and hot tubs.)

    a. _____

    b. _____

    c. _____

28. What physical changes in the elderly place them at risk for accidents?

    a. _____

    b. _____

    c. _____

    d. _____

    e. _____

29. Why should you avoid calling a person by name as a method of identifying the person?

    _____

    _____

30. When are bed rails used?

    _____

    _____

31. Box 16-3 in the textbook lists many safety measures to prevent falls. List 10 measures the support worker can do to prevent falls when giving care.

    a. _____

    b. _____

    c. _____

    d. _____

    e. _____

    f. _____

    g. _____

    h. _____

    i. _____

    j. _____

32. What safety measures can prevent burns in children?

    a. _____

    b. _____

c. _____

d. _____

e. _____

f. _____

g. _____

h. _____

i. _____

j. _____

33. What measures can help to prevent poisoning in children?

    a. _____

    b. _____

    c. _____

    d. _____

    e. _____

    f. _____

    g. _____

    h. _____

    i. _____

    j. _____

34. Children are at special risk for suffocation. What safety measures can be used to prevent suffocation in infants and children?

    a. _____

    b. _____

    c. _____

    d. _____

    e. _____

f. _____

g. _____

h. _____

i. _____

j. _____

35. List your employer's/supervisor's responsibilities under the OH&S legislation, which provides protection for you.

    a. _____

    b. _____

    c. _____

    d. _____

    e. _____

    f. _____

    g. _____

36. What are the employee's responsibilities as outlined in the OH&S legislation?

    a. _____

    b. _____

    c. _____

    d. _____

37. What are some safety measures to prevent fires?

    a. _____

    b. _____

    c. _____

    d. _____

e. _____

f. _____

38. Incident reports are used by employers and health and safety committees to _____ and

    _____.

39. Where would you find information about a hazardous substance found in the workplace?

    _____

40. What safety information should the support worker know and use when handling hazardous substances?

    a. _____

    b. _____

    c. _____

    d. _____

    e. _____

    f. _____

41. What information about hazardous materials can be found on the WHMIS label?

    a. _____

    b. _____

    c. _____

    d. _____

    e. _____

    f. _____

42. When clothing is on fire, you should _____ the person and _____ him/her with a blanket or coat to _____ the flames.

43. What personal safety measures can you take to reduce your risk of assaults?

    a. _____

    b. _____

    c. _____

    d. _____

    e. _____

    f. _____

44. How can you use your car keys as a weapon?

    _____

    _____

45. How can you use your body as a weapon if you are attacked?

    a. _____

    b. _____

    c. _____

Circle the Correct Answer

46. Bed rails are padded to
    a. prevent the person from getting caught between the rails and mattress.
    b. provide privacy for the person.
    c. prevent the person from climbing out of bed.
    d. decrease agitation.

47. What should you do if you find a smoke detector does not work in a home where you are giving care?
    a. Replace the battery
    b. Call the fire department
    c. Notify the nurse and the family
    d. This is not your responsibility—do not get involved

48. If a fire occurs, which of these steps should be done first?
    a. Use a fire extinguisher to put out the fire
    b. Close all doors and windows
    c. Sound the nearest fire alarm
    d. Move people who are in danger to a safe place

49. Suffocation can occur because
    a. a person chokes on a piece of food.
    b. a person is given a tub bath.
    c. restraints are applied correctly.
    d. dentures fit properly.

50. When an accident or error occurs, it is correct to
    a. report the accident or error immediately to your supervisor.
    b. report the incident only if a patient is injured.
    c. call the family immediately.
    d. call the doctor or ambulance.

51. If your car breaks down, a good safety practice would be to
    a. stay in the car and call police if you have a cellular phone.
    b. if someone stops to help, ask for a ride to a police station.
    c. walk to the nearest place where you can get help.
    d. get out of the car and try to flag down a ride for help.

52. If you feel uncomfortable or threatened in a home setting, you should
    a. speak to the person who is threatening you.
    b. go to a safe place immediately and call your supervisor.
    c. resign your job.
    d. have a co-worker go with you to the home.

53. Which of the following would be a threat to your safety in home care?
    a. Denial of meal breaks, drinking water, or bathroom use
    b. Inadequate heat or ventilation
    c. Being subject to name calling, obscene language
    d. All of the above

54. A person will be at increased risk of falls for all of the following factors except
    a. confusion, disorientation, and memory problems.
    b. increased joint mobility and muscle strength.
    c. visual impairment, strange surroundings, and slow reaction time.
    d. low blood pressure, dizziness on standing, and excessive alcohol use.

True or False

Circle **T** *for true or* **F** *for false. Rewrite all false statements to make them true.*

55. **T   F**   If an electric plug is not grounded, it may cause a fire.

_____

_____

56. **T   F**   Visitors need to be reminded not to smoke in a room with supplemental oxygen, even if the facility has a "No Smoking" policy.

_____

_____

57. **T   F**   Do not tie pacifiers or other items around a baby's neck.

_____

_____

58. **T   F**   Electrical equipment must be turned off before unplugging to prevent sparks.

_____

_____

59. **T   F**   Position infants on their stomach in the crib.

_____

_____

60. **T   F**   You should attempt to put out a fire before sounding a fire alarm.

_____

_____

61. **T   F**   All fire extinguishers are effective for any fire.

_____

_____

62. **T   F**   Disinfectants and cleaning solutions are hazardous substances.

_____

_____

63. **T   F**   Warnings, words, pictures, and symbols on hazardous substances may be removed after opening the container.

_____

_____

64. **T   F**   Check the MSDS after cleaning up a leak or spill, or disposing of a hazardous substance.

_____

_____

Labelling

65. What are two safety problems with the plug in the figure?

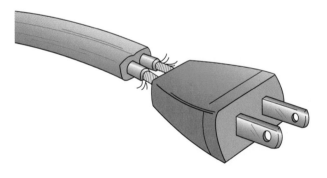

a. _____

b. _____

Independent Learning Activities

1. Safety is important to everyone and needs to be practised all the time. Check these items or areas in your own home to determine how safe your home is.
   - What areas have inadequate lighting for safety? How can the lighting be improved?
   - Check the electrical cords and plugs on appliances and lamps. How many did you discover that were frayed and damaged? What can you do to correct the unsafe cords or plugs?
   - Do you have a working smoke detector in your home? When were the batteries last changed? How often should batteries be replaced?
   - How many throw rugs are being used on a slippery surface? Do they have non-skid backing?
   - Where are medicines or household cleansers kept in your home? If they are within reach of children, where could they be placed to be out of the reach of children?
   - Make a list of the good safety practices you found in your home. Make another list of safety practices that could be improved.

2. Develop a plan for your home and family that helps everyone to escape if a fire occurs.
   - Make sure each person knows at least two escape routes from the sleeping area.
   - Practise how to check a door for heat before opening it.
   - Arrange a place to meet once you are outside of the building.

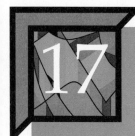

Restraint Alternatives and Safe Restraint Use

Matching

Match the description or example with the correct restraint.

1. _____ Prevents child from scratching or pulling out tubes

2. _____ A drug is given that is not required to treat the person's medical symptoms

3. _____ An attached tray keeps the person from getting up

4. _____ Hands are covered to prevent the person from removing the dressing

5. _____ May be released by the person if the quick-release type is applied

6. _____ If this is applied incorrectly, the person can strangle or suffocate

7. _____ Skin and circulation with these restraints should be checked every 15 minutes

8. _____ This type of restraint attaches a person to a nonmovable object

a. Physical restraints

b. Chemical restraint

c. Vest restraint

d. Belt restraint

e. Geriatric chair

f. Mitt restraint

g. Wrist restraint

h. Elbow restraint

True or False

*Circle **T** for true or **F** for false. Rewrite all false statements to make them true.*

9. **T F** When using restraints, the most restrictive device is used.

_____

_____

10. **T F** Apply restraint only after receiving instructions about its proper use.

_____

_____

11. **T   F**   Always follow manufacturers' instructions when using restraints.

_____

_____

12. **T   F**   Sheets, towels, or other items can be used to position a person on the toilet.

_____

_____

13. **T   F**   A vest restraint may be applied so that it crosses in either the front or the back.

_____

_____

Circle the Correct Answer

14. Which of the following statements about the use of restraints is incorrect?
    a. Unnecessary restraint is false imprisonment.
    b. People who are confused usually become calmer after being restrained.
    c. Using restraints for as little time as possible improves quality of life.
    d. The least restrictive method must be used.

15. The restraint used is determined by the
    a. doctor's order.
    b. nurse and the care plan.
    c. person applying the restraint.
    d. the legal representative.

16. Scissors should be carried when caring for people in restraints so you can
    a. trim extra long straps.
    b. remove restraints every 2 hours.
    c. remove restraints quickly in an emergency.
    d. do all of the above.

17. If you discover that a person has no pulse in a hand that is restrained, the first thing you should do is
    a. call the nurse.
    b. massage the hand.
    c. cut off the restraint.
    d. reposition the person.

18. Which of the following is *not* a risk of restraint use?
    a. Urinary and anal incontinence
    b. Bruises, nerve injuries, and pressure ulcers
    c. Increased sense of well-being and self-esteem
    d. Depression, embarrassment, humiliation, and mistrust

19. Which of these statements is *incorrect* regarding restraints?
    a. Certain drugs may be a form of restraint.
    b. Restraints may be used for staff convenience.
    c. Restraints may be used to protect a resident from harming himself/herself or others.
    d. A doctor's order is necessary for using restraints.

Fill-In-the-Blanks

20. Restraints may be used only when necessary to

_____

_____

_____

21. What are some behaviours that would allow for the use of restraints?

    a. _____

    b. _____

    c. _____

22. What is chemical restraint?

_____

_____

23. Restraints are used only when it is the

_____

_____

24. What alternatives to restraints can be used by a support worker when giving care?

a. _____

b. _____

c. _____

d. _____

e. _____

f. _____

g. _____

h. _____

i. _____

j. _____

k. _____

l. _____

25. If the support worker applies a restraint

unnecessarily, he/she could face

_____ .

26. The client or substitute decision maker must give

_____

for the use of restraints. The support worker can/cannot provide the information about restraints and obtain the signed consent.

27. When a person is restrained, the support worker must make sure basic needs are met by doing the following:

a. The person must be checked at least

_____

b. Meet the person's needs for _____ ,

_____ , _____ ,

and _____ .

28. Several staff members may be needed to apply restraints because

_____

29. Why can confusion increase when a person is restrained?

_____

_____

30. Quality of life is protected when restraints are used

for _____ .

31. How can you meet a restrained person's psychological needs?

_____

_____

32. When applying restraints, the person should be positioned in _____

and any bony areas and skin should be

_____ to

prevent _____

and _____ .

33. Restraints that are too small cause

_____

_____

_____ ,

or _____ .

34. Restraints that are too big or loose can increase the

risk of _____ .

35. If a person is restrained, what should be done at least every 2 hours?

a. _____

b. _____

c. _____

d. _____

e. _____

f. _____

36. What information should be reported to the nurse when you are caring for a restrained person?

a. _____

b. _____

c. _____

d. _____

e. _____

f. _____

g. _____

Independent Learning Activities

Role-play this situation about a client who is restrained. You and a classmate may take turns playing the roles of the client and the support worker. In order to feel as the client feels, you should be left alone for the full 20 minutes of the role playing. Use the questions to think about how you felt when you were restrained. You may think of other observations to add. After you have completed the role playing, discuss with your classmate how this situation helped to identify changes you will make when you need to restrain a client in the future.

SITUATION: Ms. Whitacre is a 92-year-old person in a nursing home. She is alert and oriented but has fallen several times when she gets up without help. The nurse tells the support worker that Ms. Whitacre needs to wear a vest restraint to keep her from falling. The support worker applies the restraint, puts Ms. Whitacre in the TV room, and leaves. Twenty minutes go by and no one comes into the TV room.

- How did you feel when the support worker said you had to be restrained?
- What did the support worker say to you when the restraint was applied? Did you understand the need for the restraint?
- How did the restraint feel on your body?
- If you had been thirsty, how would you have gotten a drink?
- How comfortable was the chair? Was the chair padded? Were you able to reposition yourself if you became tired sitting in one position?
- Were you asked if you needed to use the bathroom before the restraint was applied?
- How would you have gotten to the bathroom?
- How could you call for help? Was there a call bell in the TV room?
- Why were you in the TV room? Who decided that you would sit there? Who had control of the TV?

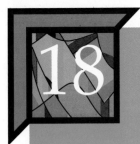

Preventing Infection

Fill-In-the-Blanks

1. What do the following statements describe?

   _____

   • They exist in five different forms.
   • They can live in a person, a plant, an animal, soil, food, water, or other material.
   • They need water, nourishment, and oxygen to live.
   • They all need a warm, dark environment to live and may be destroyed by heat and light.

2. Common reservoirs for microbes are

   _____,

   _____,

   _____,

   _____,

   _____, and

   _____.

3. The environment must be _____

   and _____ for microbes

   to survive. They also need _____

   _____ to live.

4. Why do you hold your hands down throughout the handwashing procedure?

   _____

   _____

5. Why do you turn off the water by using a paper towel to touch the hand-operated faucets?

   _____

   _____

6. What are some common signs and symptoms of a systemic infection?

   a. _____

   b. _____

   c. _____

   d. _____

   e. _____

   f. _____

   g. _____

   h. _____

   i. _____

   j. _____

7. Mr. Fox has an infection caused by a wound on his leg. How can the infection exit Mr. Fox's body?

   _____

8. How can the pathogens from Mr. Fox's infection enter another person's body?

   _____

   _____

9. What is the easiest and most important way to prevent the spread of Mr. Fox's infection?

   _____.

10. If you are wearing a gown and it becomes wet, what should you do and why?

    _____

11. Nosocomial infections are acquired _____

    _____.

12. The most common sites for nosocomial infections are

    a. _____

    b. _____

    c. _____

    d. _____

13. Nancy is a support worker caring for a person in the home. She should wash her hands

    a. _____

    b. _____

    c. _____

14. When cleaning equipment, the support worker should rinse the item in cold water first because

    _____

    _____.

15. What other guidelines should be followed when cleaning equipment?

    a. _____

    b. _____

    c. _____

    d. _____

    e. _____

16. Chemical disinfectants are used to clean

    _____.

    Utility or rubber household gloves should be worn when using a chemical disinfectant because it can

    _____.

17. An effective and cheap disinfectant for home use may be made by mixing 1 cup of

    _____ with 3 cups of

    _____.

    After preparing this solution, how should it be labelled?

    _____

18. A simple way to sterilize items in the home is to use

    _____.

19. "Standard precautions" are used to prevent the spread of infection from

    a. _____

    b. _____

    c. _____

    d. _____

20. When using standard precautions, masks, eye protection, and face shields are worn during

    _____

    _____

21. If an item is sitting on the floor, it is considered to

    be _____.

22. If you are using a sharp object when giving care, such as a razor, where should you place it when you are finished using it?

    _____

23. What part of a mask is contaminated after being worn?

_____

24. Why should you allow a person to see your face before you put on personal protective equipment?

    a. _____

    b. _____

25. What aseptic measures can the support worker use in the health care facility to control the transmission of infection?

    a. _____

    b. _____

    c. _____

    d. _____

    e. _____

    f. _____

    g. _____

26. Gloves should be changed between

_____

on the same person. Gloves should be changed

after contacting _____

_____ .

27. When you enter a room of a person with contact precautions, you should wear

_____ .

You should change your

_____

after having contact with

_____ .

28. When you are assigned to care for a person in isolation you should tell the nurse if you have any

_____ .

29. What are some of the rules to follow when caring for a client under transmission-based precautions?

    a. _____

    b. _____

    c. _____

    d. _____

    e. _____

30. What are some examples of sharps containers that may be used in home care?

    a. _____

    b. _____

    c. _____

    d. _____

31. When you care for a client with an infection, what precautions should be used when handling contaminated laundry?

    a. _____

    b. _____

    c. _____

    d. _____

    e. _____

Circle the Correct Answer

32. When you contaminate your hands while working in a health care facility, you should wash your hands for at least
    a. 3 to 5 minutes.
    b. 2 minutes.
    c. 15 to 20 seconds.
    d. 1 minute.

33. Which of these statements is *not* a good aseptic measure?
    a. Do not take clean, unused equipment from one person's room to another room
    b. Clean from the dirtiest area to the cleanest
    c. Wear protective equipment as needed
    d. Keep tables and other surfaces clean and dry

34. Here is a list of common aseptic practices that you should use. Which one is the most important to prevent the spread of infection?
    a. Bathing, washing hair, and brushing teeth regularly
    b. Washing cooking utensils with soap and water
    c. Covering nose and mouth when coughing or sneezing
    d. Washing hands immediately before and after client care as necessary

35. Transmission-based precautions are used when caring
    a. for all persons.
    b. for persons with open wounds.
    c. depending on how the pathogen is spread.
    d. only for persons with a respiratory infection.

36. When you are caring for a person who is in isolation, what should you do if you drop clean linens on the floor?
    a. Pick them up and return them to the stack of clean linens
    b. They are contaminated and should be thrown in the trash
    c. They are contaminated and should be placed in the dirty linen container
    d. Use them immediately so they are mixed with clean linens

37. Paper towels are used in isolation
    a. to handle contaminated items.
    b. under clean items or objects.
    c. to turn faucets on and off.
    d. for all of the above.

38. Standard precautions should be used
    a. only when you think a person has an infection.
    b. only when you are changing soiled linens.
    c. only when you have open skin wounds.
    d. when caring for all persons at all times.

39. When you are removing gloves after giving care, which part is considered "clean?"
    a. The inside
    b. The outside
    c. Both sides
    d. Neither side

40. When transporting a person who is in isolation, the person should wear a mask
    a. at all times.
    b. until the person reaches the destination.
    c. if the person is on airborne or droplet precautions.
    d. only on an elevator.

41. Which of the following aseptic measures will control the portal of entry?
    a. Make sure all persons have their own personal care equipment
    b. Make sure drainage tubes are correctly connected
    c. Cover your nose and mouth when coughing or sneezing
    d. Keep drainage containers below drainage sites

42. If a container is labelled "biohazard," it contains materials that are
    a. sterile.
    b. clean.
    c. contaminated.
    d. poisonous.

43. Which, if any, of these gloves can be reused after cleaning?
    a. Sterile gloves
    b. Disposable gloves
    c. Utility gloves
    d. None of the above

44. Which of the following statements about wearing gloves is *incorrect?*
    a. Remove and discard torn or punctured gloves immediately
    b. Wear the same gloves when giving care to both people in a semiprivate room
    c. Put on clean gloves just before touching mucous membranes or nonintact skin
    d. Wash your hands after removing gloves

45. When is double bagging of biohazardous waste necessary?
    a. Any time contaminated items are removed from the person's room
    b. When the person has contact precautions
    c. When materials are contaminated with body fluids
    d. When the outside of the biohazard bag has been contaminated

46. When putting on sterile gloves, which of the following steps is correct?
    a. Lift the second glove by touching only the inside of the glove
    b. Pick up the first glove by reaching under the cuff with your hand
    c. Hold the thumb of your first gloved hand away from your second hand as you put on the glove
    d. Place the glove package below waist height

47. How can you help to prevent a decrease in self-esteem when a person is in isolation?
    a. Discourage visits by family and friends
    b. Maintain distance between you and the person
    c. Arrange to spend time to visit with the person
    d. Remain in the room only for a short time

Matching

Match the practice used in transmission-based precautions with the correct type of precaution. (Some precautions may have more than one answer.)

48. _____ Do not enter room of person with measles or chickenpox if you are susceptible to these diseases

49. _____ Wear a mask when working within 1 m of the person

50. _____ Wear gloves when entering the room

51. _____ Keep the door of the room closed

52. _____ Wear a gown on entering the room if the person is incontinent or has diarrhea

53. _____ Wear tuberculosis respirator when entering room of person with known or suspected tuberculosis

54. _____ Wash your hands immediately with an agent specified by the nurse in charge

a. Airborne precautions

b. Droplet precautions

c. Contact precautions

True or False

Circle T for true or F for false. Rewrite all false statements to make them true.

55. T   F   Microbes get oxygen and nourishment from the reservoir.

_____

_____

56. T   F   Microbes are destroyed by a warm, dark environment.

_____

_____

57. T   F   Items can be sterilized in the home with boiling water.

_____

_____

58. T   F   If you must transport a person who has an infection that requires droplet or airborne precautions out of his/her room, the person must wear a disposable gown.

_____

_____

59. **T** **F** When you remove gloves, the inside is considered clean.

_____

_____

60. **T** **F** If a sterile item touches a clean item, the sterile item is contaminated.

_____

_____

61. **T** **F** If a clean item touches a sterile item, the clean item is contaminated.

_____

_____

62. **T** **F** If a sterile item is above your waist, it is contaminated.

_____

_____

Diagrams

63. Identify the parts of the hands that are frequently missed during handwashing.

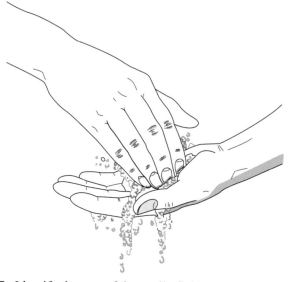

64. Identify the part of the gown that is considered contaminated after use.

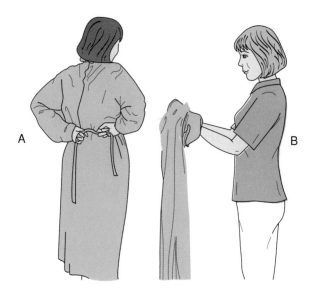

A   B

67. Identify the part of the sterile field that is considered contaminated.

Independent Learning Activities

1. Handwashing is an important practice to prevent the spread of infection. Make a list for 1 day (away from school or work) of the times and places you wash your hands. At the end of the day make a second list of times you should have washed your hands and did not. How can you improve your handwashing practice? How have your handwashing habits changed since studying this chapter?

2. When you are working in a health care facility, you need to prevent the spread of infection. Use the situation to identify ways to prevent spreading disease. Consider how you would answer these questions about caring for Mr. Gonzalez.

   SITUATION: Mr. Gonzalez, 50, is admitted to the facility. He is placed under contact precautions.
   - What are the body fluids you are going to handle carefully?
   - How can you protect yourself against infection in this situation? What will you wear?
   - How will you dispose of vomitus? stool? urine? respiratory secretions?
   - How will you handle soiled tissues lying on the floor?
   - What items will need to be labelled "biohazard" when being removed from the room?
   - What would you do if Mr. Gonzalez cut himself while shaving?
   - What would you do if you cut your leg on the bed while working in this room?

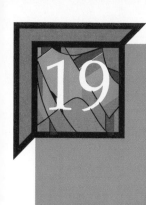

19

Abuse

Matching

Match the correct terms with their definitions.

1. ___e___ Failure to meet basic needs   a. Sexual abuse

2. ___d___ Misuse of a person's money   b. Physical abuse

3. ___b___ Force or violence that causes injury   c. Emotional abuse

4. ___a___ Unwanted sexual activity   d. Financial abuse

5. ___c___ Words or actions that inflict mental harm   e. Neglect

Match the different forms of client abuse with the appropriate description.

6. ___b___ Threatening punishment or deprival of needs   a. Physical

7. ___a___ Inflicting punishment on the body   b. Violation of rights

8. ___c___ Harassing or attacking a person sexually   c. Sexual

9. ___d___ Person's money is used by another person without consent   d. Financial

10. ___e___ Providing care against the person's wishes   e. Emotional

True or False

*Circle **T** for true or **F** for false. Rewrite all false statements to make them true.*

11. **T   F**   Usually the time between abusive events gradually shortens.

_____

_____

12. **T   F**   More women are abused by spouses than males.

_____

_____

13. **T   F**   People who are abused often deny the abuse.

_____

_____

14. **T   F**   Slapping a child is not considered abuse.

_____

_____

15. **T   F**   Emotional and physical abuse are the most common types of abuse of older adults.

_____

_____

16. **T   F**   Ageism is another cause of abuse.

_____

_____

17. **T   F**   Failing to provide privacy is not a form of abuse.

_____

_____

18. **T   F**   Changes in mental function can cause someone to become sexually abusive.

_____

_____

19. **T   F**   Masturbation may be the result of urinary problems in a confused resident.

_____

_____

20. **T   F**   The best way to handle someone who is masturbating in public is to tell the person to stop.

_____

_____

21. **T   F**   You are legally responsible to report child abuse and (in some juristictions) abuse within facilities.

_____

_____

22. **T   F**   Sexual harassment is not considered sexual abuse.

_____

_____

23. **T   F**   Abuse is usually triggered by an event related to the victim.

_____

_____

24. **T   F**   People who were abused as children are not likely to abuse their own children because they know what it was like.

_____

_____

25. **T F** In most provinces, you do not have to report abuse of older adults to a public authority if it occurs in home care settings.

_____

_____

Circle the Correct Answer

26. If you suspect a person is being abused, you should
    a. call the police.
    b. talk to the family.
    c. report it to an RN.
    d. talk to the person being abused.

27. If you are dealing with an agitated or aggressive person, which of these measures would be most helpful?
    a. Talk to the person in a calm manner
    b. Place your hand on the person's arm to prevent injury
    c. Close the door so that other people are not upset
    d. Promise the person you will not tell anyone else about his/her behaviour

Fill-In-the-Blanks

28. The three phases in the cycle of abuse are
    a. _Tension Building phase_
    b. _Abusive Phase_
    c. _honey moon "_

29. A person is more likely to be abusive if he or she
    a. _has problems w/ alcohol or drugs_
    b. _has mental illness or severe personality flaws_
    c. _has been abused as child_
    d. _is going under the period of high stress_

30. Certain situations increase the risk of child abuse. They are
    a. _family crisis_
    b. _single parenting_
    c. _isolation_
    d. _caring for children w/ special need_

31. Why do abused older adults choose not to complain about the abuse?
    a. _fear of abuser_
    b. _not wanting to a long-term facility_
    c. _____
    d. _____

32. Examples of how workers might abuse clients in a facility or home are
    a. _____
    b. _____
    c. _____
    d. _____
    e. _____
    f. _____

33. What are some examples of abuse that a support worker may encounter from clients?
    a. _____
    b. _____
    c. _____
    d. _____
    e. _____

34. What can you do when a client is being abusive?

a. _____

b. _____

c. _____

d. _____

e. _____

f. _____

35 Give three signs/symptoms of each type of abuse.

Physical abuse

a. _____

b. _____

c. _____

Sexual abuse

a. _____

b. _____

c. _____

Emotional abuse

a. _____

b. _____

c. _____

Financial abuse

a. _____

b. _____

c. _____

Neglect

a. _____

b. _____

c. _____

36. What should you do if a client tells you that he/she is being abused?

a. _____

b. _____

c. _____

d. _____

e. _____

37. Name the types of child abuse described in the examples below.

A welt in the shape of a belt buckle is found on the body.

a. _____

A child is kissed, touched, or fondled inappropriately.

b. _____

A child is deprived of food and clothing.

c. _____

A child is forced to engage in sexual activity for money.

d. _____

A child's need for affection and attention is not met.

e. _____

A child is threatened and called names.

f. _____

*For each of these situations, identify what tort has been committed. Then circle **I** for intentional or **U** for unintentional.*

38. **I   U** _____

While cleaning a person's dentures, the support worker drops and breaks them.

39. **I   U** _____

A support worker opens a person's mail and reads it.

40. **I   U** _____

Instead of allowing the person a choice, the support worker tells the person that he/she will get a shower whether or not he/she wants one.

41. **I   U** _____

A person put on the signal light 20 minutes ago. The person tries to go to the bathroom alone, slips and falls, and breaks a hip.

42. **I   U** _____

A support worker talks to employees from other departments about a client.

43. **I   U** _____

After her morning care is completed, a client wants to go to do activities. The support worker does not allow the client to go.

44. **I   U** _____

An individual has failed to act in a reasonable and careful manner and caused harm to the person or property of another.

45. **I   U** _____

An individual has injured the name and reputation of a person by making false statements to a third person.

46. **I   U** _____

An individual attempts or threatens to touch another person's body without the person's consent.

47. **I   U** _____

An individual touches another person's body without the person's consent.

48. **I   U** _____

An individual exposes the private affairs of another person to a third person.

49. **I   U** _____

An individual tricks or fools another person.

50. **I   U** _____

An individual restrains or restricts another person's freedom of movement without a physician's order.

Independent Learning Activities

Consider this situation about a sexually aggressive person, and answer the questions about how you would respond.

SITUATION: Mr. James is 72 and has paraplegia because of an accident that occurred several years ago. His caregivers report that recently he has begun to make sexually suggestive remarks. While you are giving him his a.m. care, he keeps touching you in private areas and makes frequent sexually suggestive remarks. The other support workers tell you that they just ignore him or joke around with him about the actions.
- What would you say to Mr. James when he touched you in private areas?
- How would you respond to his suggestive remarks?
- What would you say to your colleagues who suggest that you ignore or joke with Mr. James?
- Has this type of situation ever occurred to you? How did you handle it then? What would you do differently after studying this chapter?

20

The Client's Environment: Promoting Well-Being, Comfort, and Rest

Matching

Match the comfort factors with the actions that the support worker can take to control these factors.

1. _____ Adjusting the thermostat in the room

2. _____ Turning lights down during rest periods

3. _____ Emptying bedpans and urinals promptly

4. _____ Washing hands after smoking

5. _____ Opening windows and doors and turning on fans as client desires

6. _____ Making sure person has good personal care

7. _____ Talking quietly to staff members

8. _____ Opening shades or drapes when person is reading

a. Temperature

b. Ventilation

c. Noise

d. Odours

e. Lighting

True or False

*Circle **T** for true or **F** for false. Rewrite all false statements to make them true.*

9. **T   F**   Personal items in a person's unit are arranged as the individual prefers.

_____

_____

10. **T   F**   The support worker may throw away any items in the person's unit that are in the way.

_____

_____

11. **T   F**   Make sure the person can reach the telephone, television, and light controls.

_____

_____

12. **T   F**   Moving furniture or belongings may be a safety hazard for a person with poor vision.

_____

_____

Circle the Correct Answer

13. The call bell should always be positioned
    a. on the bed rail.
    b. attached to the pillow.
    c. within the person's reach.
    d. on the arm of the chair.

14. If you wish to locate an item in a person's closet, you should
    a. wait until he/she is out of the room to search.
    b. tell him/her that you must find the item and begin to search.
    c. ask his/her permission to look for the item.
    d. inform the nurse and have her/him look for the item.

15. You are admitting a new person. Which of these situations should be reported to the nurse immediately?
    a. The person complains of pain and appears to be in distress.
    b. The person cries and expresses a desire to go home.
    c. The person has difficulty hearing you.
    d. Both a and b above.

16. Mrs. Smith is being admitted to a facility. She wants a family member to stay with her during the admission process. What should you do?
    a. Tell the family member he/she must leave.
    b. Tell the nurse.
    c. Understand that this is a critical and emotional time for Mrs. Smith and her family, and let the family member stay.
    d. Address all questions to the family member because he/she can answer more quickly than Mrs. Smith can.

17. Which of the following tasks is a support worker's responsibility when discharging a person?
    a. Packing the person's belongings
    b. Teaching the person about a new diet
    c. Making the person an appointment with the doctor
    d. Teaching the person about dressing changes

Fill-In-the-Blanks

18. If a person complains of pain, the person:

_____ .

19. What type of pain is felt suddenly from injury, disease, trauma, or surgery?

_____

20. How do these factors affect pain?

a. Past experience

_____

b. Anxiety

_____

c. Rest and sleep

_____

d. Attention

_____

e. Value or meaning of pain

_____

f. Support from others

_____

g. Culture

_____

h. Age

_____

21. The nurse needs certain information to assess the person's pain. What questions could you ask to help gather this information for the nurse?

    a. Location _____

    _____

    b. Onset and duration _____

    _____

    c. Intensity _____

    _____

    d. Description _____

    _____

    e. Factors causing pain _____

    _____

    f. Vital signs _____

    _____

    g. Other signs and symptoms _____

    _____

22. What reaction to pain may occur with a person from these cultures?

    a. Philippines _____

    _____

    b. Vietnam _____

    _____

    c. China _____

    _____

23. Why are older people at greater risk for undetected disease or injury?

    _____

24. What body responses may be signs and symptoms of pain?

    a. _____

    b. _____

    c. _____

    d. _____

    e. _____

25. What are some of the safety measures used when the person is receiving strong pain medications?

    a. _____

    b. _____

    c. _____

    d. _____

26. How long should you wait to perform procedures after pain medications are given?

    _____

27. The nurse asks you to assist with these measures to control pain. What is done with each one?

    a. Distraction _____

    _____

    b. Relaxation _____

    _____

    c. Guided imagery _____

    _____

28. When a person experiences pain, it cannot be seen, heard, felt, or smelled. How can you know the person has pain?

    _____

29. What are some ways you may be able to tell that an infant or young child has pain?

    _____

30. Ill or injured people need to rest more often. How can you help them to get the rest needed?

_____

31. What would be the average amount of sleep these people would require per day?

a. 6-month-old infant _____

_____

b. 5-year-old boy _____

_____

c. 17-year-old girl _____

_____

d. 35-year-old man _____

_____

e. 65-year-old woman _____

_____

32. What foods or liquids can help sleep?

_____

33. How do the following factors affect sleep?

a. Illness _____

_____

b. Nutrition _____

_____

c. Exercise at bedtime _____

_____

d. Environment _____

_____

e. Medications and alcohol _____

_____

f. Changes and stress _____

_____

g. Emotional problems _____

_____

34. What can you do to the person's room to promote sleep?

a. _____

b. _____

c. _____

d. _____

35. What drinks should be avoided before going to bed?

a. _____

b. _____

36. List ways that a homelike environment can be provided in a long-term care facility.

a. _____

b. _____

c. _____

d. _____

37. Higher room temperatures will probably be needed by persons in these age groups.

a. _____

b. _____

38. Why are toilets in some health care facilities higher than standard toilets?

a. _____

b. _____

39. How can you help a new resident and family feel comfortable, safe, and secure during the admission procedure?

    Offer them _____

    _____ .

    Introduce them to _____

    _____ .

    Help resident to hang _____

    _____ .

40. Who is responsible for explaining to the person the reasons for a transfer to another room, nursing unit, or facility?

    _____

    _____

41. When you transfer a person to a new unit, what should you tell the receiving nurse?

    a. _____

    b. _____

42. What should you do if a person expresses an intent to leave the facility without the doctor's permission?

    _____

    _____

Matching

Match the type of pain with the correct description.

43. _____ Pain is felt at the site of tissue damage and in nearby areas

44. _____ Pain is felt suddenly and lasts a short time

45. _____ Pain is felt in a body part that is no longer there

46. _____ Pain lasts longer than 6 months

a. Acute pain

b. Chronic pain

c. Radiating pain

d. Phantom pain

Match the words below to a behaviour or descriptive word related to pain.

47. _____ Aching

48. _____ Throbbing

49. _____ Groaning

50. _____ Restlessness

51. _____ Squeezing

52. _____ Knifelike

53. _____ Dull

54. _____ Irritability

55. _____ Quietness

a. Behaviour that is a sign or symptom of pain

b. Words used to describe

Circle the Correct Answer

56. Which of the following statements about pain is *not* true?
    a. Pain is different for each person.
    b. Pain is easy to measure with objective assessments.
    c. Pain means there is damage to body tissue.
    d. You must rely on the person to tell you about the pain.

57. Which of the following statements does *not* describe chronic pain?
    a. Pain lasts longer than 6 months.
    b. Pain is felt at the site and in nearby areas.
    c. Pain may be constant or occur off and on.
    d. Pain remains long after healing occurs.

58. What type of pain occurs when a person has an amputated leg and still feels pain in the missing limb?
    a. Acute
    b. Chronic
    c. Radiating
    d. Phantom

59. If a person is unable to fall asleep, is unable to stay asleep, or awakens easily and cannot fall back to sleep, the person
    a. has sleep deprivation.
    b. has insomnia.
    c. is sleepwalking.
    d. has emotional problems.

Independent Learning Activities

1. Organize a group discussion with three or four classmates to share your personal experiences with pain. Answer the questions to understand differences in pain perception and management.
   - What experiences have you had with pain? Accidents? Illness? Childbirth? Surgery?
   - How long did your pain last? What type of pain was it? Chronic? Acute?
   - How would you rate the pain on a scale of 1 to 10?
   - How did your family, friends, and others respond to your pain? How did you feel about their responses?
   - How did you deal with the pain? What measures did you use to relieve the pain?
   - How will this discussion about personal experience with pain affect your approach to a person who has pain?

2. Use this situation to explore your responsibilities when caring for a person who is being transferred within a facility.
   SITUATION: Ms. Beauchemin, 55, had surgery for a knee replacement last week. She is recovering well but is having trouble going up and down stairs independently. She needs further exercise before going home because her house has two floors and she lives alone. She is being transferred to a rehabilitation unit, and you are assigned to assist her. Answer the following questions about your responsibility in transferring a person within a health care facility.
   - What would you say to Ms. Beauchemin when you went to her room? What would you do if she seemed unaware that a transfer were planned? Who would be responsible for telling her about the move?
   - What would you do to help Ms. Beauchemin prepare for the move? What would you need to do to make sure that all her belongings were moved? What equipment would you need to transport her and her belongings to the new unit?
   - When you and Ms. Beauchemin arrive at the rehabilitation unit, what should you do first? What information would you need to give to the receiving nurse?
   - What other responsibilities would you need to carry out after your return?

   SITUATION: Two weeks have passed since Ms. Beauchemin was transferred to the rehabilitation unit. When you arrive at work, you are sent to the rehabilitation unit for the day. You find that you are assigned to assist Ms. Beauchemin, and she is being discharged today. Answer these questions about your responsibilities in discharging a person from a health care facility.
   - What information should you check before going to Ms. Beauchemin's room? Where would you find this information?
   - How would you make sure that you had gathered all of Ms. Beauchemin's clothing and her belongings? What should you have Ms. Beauchemin do in order to document that all of her clothing has been returned to her?
   - When you leave the unit with Ms. Beauchemin, where would you take her for discharge?
   - What would you report to the nurse when you returned to the unit? What other responsibilities would you have to carry out after the discharge?

3. Check the temperature in your home. People have different temperatures at which they are comfortable. Answer these questions about yourself to help you understand the importance of individual preferences for people in a health care setting.
   - Do you prefer hot or cold rooms? Why?
   - How does the temperature that you prefer compare with that of your spouse, children, or friends?
   - Would the temperature you prefer be appropriate for an infant? An older adult? Why or why not?

4. How does noise in your home affect you? Answer these questions to help you understand the importance of noise levels in the health care facility.
   - How do you study best? With the radio or TV on? With silence?
   - When you go to bed, do you prefer silence to help you to sleep? Do you like the sound of soft music or the TV as you go to sleep?
   - Does everyone in your household agree on what volume to keep the radio or TV? How do you resolve conflict over this if it is a problem?
   - If the noise level in your surroundings is unacceptable to you, how do you react? How does it affect your ability to think? Rest? Study? How does it affect your relationship with others?

21

Body Mechanics: Moving, Positioning, and Transferring the Client

Word Search

Write the correct word next to each definition on the following page. Find each word in the Word Search and mark (circle, highlight, or draw line through) the words.

A	B	O	D	Y	M	E	C	H	A	N	P	S	I	T	S
C	O	J	D	E	O	L	S	L	A	T	E	R	A	L	P
Z	Y	E	R	A	O	Q	T	O	D	D	R	A	O	O	R
L	F	R	A	R	W	U	M	G	N	T	A	I	T	N	I
O	R	O	W	S	H	E	A	R	I	N	G	N	H	O	E
L	I	T	S	Z	I	S	T	O	M	G	A	K	G	A	L
T	C	A	H	Y	U	M	O	L	V	T	I	L	O	L	M
S	T	E	E	P	L	T	S	L	O	A	T	E	A	I	E
O	I	L	E	S	R	Y	V	I	O	N	B	I	N	G	L
P	O	S	T	U	R	E	S	N	N	W	E	B	A	N	T
O	N	T	O	P	O	F	T	G	E	T	L	V	O	M	Z
P	F	O	L	I	N	O	L	I	R	X	T	M	E	E	T
U	R	R	O	N	C	F	O	W	L	E	R	S	O	N	P
P	Y	W	H	E	E	L	C	H	A	I	R	B	O	T	E

1. _____ Rubbing of one surface against another

2. _____ Way in which body parts are aligned with one another

3. _____ When the skin sticks to a surface and the muscles slide in the direction the body is moving

4. _____ Transfer or safety belt

5. _____ Turning the person as a unit in alignment in one motion

6. _____ Back-lying or dorsal recumbent position

7. _____ Side-lying position

8. _____ Semi-sitting position with head of bed elevated 45 to 60 degrees

9. _____ Side-lying position in which upper leg is sharply flexed

10. _____ Another word for posture; body _____

11. _____ A lift sheet; a turn or pull sheet

12. _____ Sit on the edge of the bed

13. _____ Position on abdomen with head turned to one side

14. _____ Chair used to move person from one place to another

Fill-In-the-Blanks

15. It is important for a support worker to follow the guidelines for good body mechanics. They are

    a. _____

    b. _____

    c. _____

    d. _____

    e. _____

    f. _____

    g. _____

    h. _____

16. How can you provide a better base of support for yourself when lifting?

    _____

17. Providing a good base of support will help to reduce the risk of _____ .

18. When you move a person up in bed, it is important to protect the skin from _____ .

19. When moving a person up in bed, why should you place the pillow against the headboard?

    _____

20. How can you provide comfort and safety to a person being lifted or moved in bed?

    a. _____

    b. _____

    c. _____

    d. _____

    e. _____

    f. _____

21. Why should the level of the bed be raised horizontally when the person is being repositioned?

    _____

22. Why should two staff members work together when raising an older person's head and shoulders?

    _____

23. How can you make sure that you and a co-worker both move the person at the same time when working together?

    _____

24. When a lift sheet is used _____ and _____ are reduced, the person can be _____ .

25. Why should you move a person to the side of the bed before turning?

    _____

26. Logrolling is used to turn

    a. _____

    b. _____

    c. _____

    d. _____

27. What observations should you make when the person is dangling?

    a. _____

    b. _____

    c. _____

    d. _____

    e. _____

    f. _____

    g. _____

28. A transfer belt is used to transfer

    _____ and

    _____ people.

29. How many staff members are needed to transfer a person from the bed to a chair or wheelchair?

    _____

30. Why do you pad the seat of the wheelchair?

    _____

    _____

31. When are mechanical lifts used?

    _____

    _____

32. Before using a lift, make sure

    a. _____

    b. _____

    c. _____

33. When you position a person, you should follow these safety regulations:

    a. _____

    b. _____

    c. _____

    d. _____

    e. _____

    f. _____

    g. _____

    h. _____

    i. _____

34. What are the benefits of repositioning a person frequently?

    a. _____

    b. _____

    c. _____

    d. _____

True or False

Circle **T** *for true or* **F** *for false. Rewrite all false statements to make them true.*

35. **T** **F**   Logrolling keeps the spine straight.

_____

_____

36. **T** **F**   When you lift, move, or carry objects, hold them with arms extended.

_____

_____

37. **T** **F**   When lifting an object from the floor, bend from the waist.

_____

_____

38. **T** **F**   Using two or more people to move a heavy, weak, or very old person up in bed protects only the person from injury.

_____

_____

39. **T** **F**   A lift sheet or turning sheet can be a folded sheet, draw sheet, or turning pad.

_____

_____

40. **T** **F**   When transferring a person to a chair, you should be primarily concerned that the chair is comfortable.

_____

_____

41. **T** **F**   Repositioning of a person lying in bed or sitting in a chair should be done every 3 to 4 hours.

_____

_____

Circle the Correct Answer

42. A lift sheet is used by placing the sheet under the person
    a. from the head to above the knees.
    b. from the shoulders to the hips.
    c. from the head to the hips.
    d. from the shoulders to the knees.

43. Why should shoes with nonskid soles be worn by the person being transferred to a chair or wheelchair?
    a. Provide good base of support
    b. Make person more steady on his/her feet
    c. Prevent sliding or slipping on floor
    d. Provide strength on the person's weak side

44. When transferring a person to a stretcher,
    a. three or more staff members are needed.
    b. a transfer belt is used to lift the person.
    c. the head of the stretcher is raised before the transfer.
    d. the person is transported head first.

Labelling

Label the basic positions illustrated.

45. The position is _____.

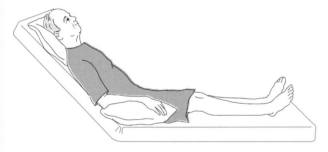

46. The position is _____.

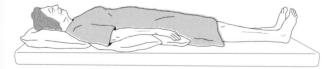

47. The position is _____
    with a pillow placed under the _____
    _____
    to prevent pressure on the toes.

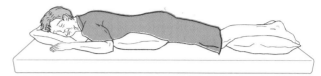

48. The position is _____
    with the feet positioned over
    _____
    _____.

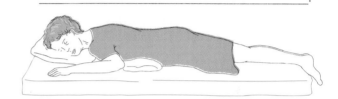

49. The position is _____.

50. The position is _____.

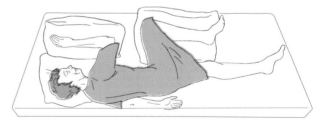

51. When lifting correctly, which muscles are used?

_____

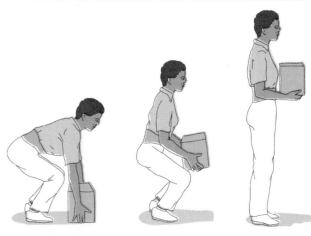

Independent Learning Activities

1. For 1 day, pay attention to how well you use body mechanics in your daily life. When did you use correct methods to prevent strain or injury? When could you have used body mechanics better?

   Consider if you had performed the following actions:
   - Lifting textbooks by bending your knees rather than bending your back
   - Carrying garbage to the garbage can holding it close to your body
   - Carrying groceries into the house holding the bags close to your body
   - Making two or more trips when carrying items rather than trying to carry too much at once

2. Role-play this situation with a classmate. Take turns acting as Mr. Green and as the support worker. Have a third classmate act as an observer to tell each of you when you used good body mechanics and when you did not.

   SITUATION: Mr. Green is a 78-year-old man who had a stroke (CVA, brain attack) last month. He has paralysis on his right side. The nurse asks you to turn him from his back to his left side and position him comfortably.
   - How can you turn Mr. Green to prevent injury to him?
   - What assistive devices could you use? How would they be helpful?
   - How many pillows are needed for comfort and good alignment?
   - When you are playing Mr. Green, how does it feel to be moved by someone else?
   - After you are positioned, are you comfortable?
   - How can you signal the nurse or support worker, answer the phone, or get a drink of water in this position?

3. Role play this situation with two classmates. Take turns acting as Ms. Simpson and as the support worker. Be sure you do not place weight on your right leg when you are Ms. Simpson.

   SITUATION: Ms. Simpson, 72, fell in the hall and injured her right leg. She needs to be transported by wheelchair to x-ray. You are assigned to get her ready to go. Consider these questions to determine how you will safely move Ms. Simpson.
   - How will you prepare Ms. Simpson for the transfer? What will you tell her? What clothing should she wear?
   - How will you prepare the wheelchair? Safety preparation? Comfort concerns?
   - On which side of the bed will you position the wheelchair? Why?
   - What assessments of Ms. Simpson are likely to be done before and after the transfer? Why?
   - What factors would determine whether you will use a transfer belt or not?
   - How will you position yourself as you prepare to transfer Ms. Simpson?
   - How will you move to prevent injury to yourself?

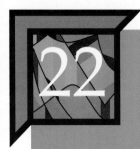

Exercise and Activity

Matching

Match the following statements with the correct term related to exercise and activity.

1. _____ Supports placed to prevent external rotation of hips and legs

2. _____ Swinging bar on overbed frame that allows person to move in bed

3. _____ Decrease in size or wasting away of tissue

4. _____ Turning downward

5. _____ Device placed to keep soles of feet flush against it with feet in flexed position

6. _____ Abnormal shortening of a muscle

7. _____ Sections of plywood used to prevent mattress from sagging

8. _____ Foot drop

9. _____ Exercise of all joints of the body

a. Foot board

b. Contracture

c. Atrophy

d. Bed board

e. Plantar flexion

f. Trochanter roll

g. Trapeze

h. Range-of-motion

i. Pronation

Match each movement with the description.

10. _____ Turn head from side to side

11. _____ Turn hand so palm is down

12. _____ Turn hand toward thumb

13. _____ Bend arm so that same-side shoulder is touched

14. _____ Pull foot forward and push down on heel at same time

15. _____ Move straight arm away from side of body

16. _____ Turn foot down or point the toes

a. Abduction

b. Adduction

c. Flexion

d. Internal rotation

e. Extension

f. Hyperextension

g. Rotation

17. _____ Move head to the right and to the left

18. _____ Touch each fingertip to thumb

19. _____ Turn hand toward little finger

20. _____ Move forearm toward head

21. _____ Move leg toward the other leg

22. _____ Straighten fingers so fingers, hand, and wrist are straight

23. _____ Bend the hand back

24. _____ Turn inside of foot up and outside down

25. _____ Turn leg inward

h. Lateral flexion

i. External rotation

j. Pronation

k. Supination

l. Opposition

m. Plantar flexion

n. Dorsiflexion

o. Radial flexion

p. Ulnar flexion

Fill-In-the-Blanks

26. Describe the following types of bed rest:

    a. Bed rest

    _____

    b. Strict bed rest

    _____

    c. Bed rest with commode privileges

    _____

    d. Bed rest with bathroom privileges

    _____

27. What are the benefits of bedrest?

    a. _____

    b. _____

    c. _____

    d. _____

    e. _____

28. What problem can be prevented by using a foot board?

    _____

29. What device can be used to prevent external rotation of the hips and legs?

    _____

30. What is the purpose of a hip abduction wedge and where is it positioned?

    _____

31. Depending on the child's activity limits, almost any play activity promotes

    _____ in children.

32. Describe the following types of range-of-motion exercises:

    a. Active

    _____

    b. Passive

    _____

    c. Active-assistive

    _____

33. What device is used to safely transfer or ambulate the person?

    _____

34. Why do you ease a person who is falling onto the floor instead of trying to stop the fall?

   _____

35. On which side of the body is the cane used when ambulating?

   _____

36. A person using a cane should follow these steps.

   a. Step A

   _____

   b. Step B

   _____

   c. Step C

   _____

37. Why do some people prefer a walker to a cane?

   _____

38. How far in front of the person is a walker moved with each step?

   _____

Circle the Correct Answer

39. Which of the following statements correctly describes a type of bed rest?
   a. Person remains in bed, but some ADL are allowed
   b. Person can use the bedside commode for elimination needs
   c. Everything is done for the person; no ADLs are allowed
   d. All of the above describe bed rest

40. Which of the following steps would not be used to prevent orthostatic hypotension?
   a. Assist the person to sit on the edge of the bed
   b. Ask the person about weakness, dizziness, or spots before the eyes
   c. Have the person stand up quickly when getting out of bed
   d. Measure blood pressure, pulse, and respirations each time the person changes position

41. Which of the following is *not* a complication of bed rest?
   a. Urinary incontinence
   b. Constipation
   c. Blood clots
   d. Pneumonia

42. What is one range-of-motion exercise that is done only if allowed by the agency?
   a. Hip abduction and adduction
   b. Neck exercises
   c. Knee exercises
   d. Shoulder exercises

43. When you move a joint during range-of-motion exercises and the person complains of pain, what should you do?
   a. Ask the nurse to give pain medication before you continue
   b. Do not force the joint to the point of pain
   c. Stop giving any range-of-motion exercises
   d. Push slightly past the point where pain occurs to restore movement

44. When performing range-of-motion exercises, how often should each exercise be repeated?
   a. Once
   b. Twice
   c. Five times or according to the plan of care
   d. Until the person complains of being tired

45. Improperly fitted crutches can cause
   a. falls.
   b. back pain and nerve damage.
   c. injuries to the underarms and palms.
   d. all of the above.

True or False

Circle T *for true or* F *for false. Rewrite all false statements to make them true.*

46. T F Exercise every joint on every person.

   _____

   _____

47. T F Support the extremity being exercised.

   _____

   _____

48. **T   F**   Exercise the joint to the point of pain.

_____

_____

49. **T   F**   The person should wear soft slippers or sandals when using crutches.

_____

_____

50. **T   F**   Loose clothing can hang forward and block the person's view of the feet and crutches.

_____

_____

51. **T   F**   A pouch attached to a walker makes the person more dependent on others.

_____

_____

Labelling

52. Identify the movements shown in each image.

a. _____

_____

_____

b. _____

_____

c. _____

_____

53. Identify the movements shown.

a. _____

b. _____

Independent Learning Activities

1. With a classmate, role-play this situation with each of you taking a turn playing Mrs. Beall.

   SITUATION: Mrs. Beall is 85 and is very weak. She needs assistance to get out of bed, stand up, and walk. You are assigned to assist her to ambulate in the hall using a walker or her cane. As you walk down the hall, Mrs. Beall tells you she feels weak and faint. She loses her balance and begins to fall.

   Answer these questions to help you understand how a person may feel when needing assistance with walking.
   - What was Mrs. Beall told before the ambulation exercise began? What did she know about the distance planned, the assistance that would be given, and what she needed to do?
   - How did the choice of clothing provide comfort and safety? What type of shoes and clothing was she wearing? What opportunity did Mrs. Beall have to choose her clothing?
   - What other steps were taken to provide for safety? What devices were used to prevent falls? What steps were taken to check the walker or cane for safety?
   - What assessments were made when she first sat on the edge of the bed?
   - When you were Mrs. Beall, how secure did you feel when you were being ambulated? How did the support worker make you feel you were safe? When you were the support worker, how secure did you feel about keeping Mrs. Beall safe?
   - What methods did you use to hold her securely?
   - As the support worker, what did you do when Mrs. Beall lost her balance? What techniques did you use to prevent injury to Mrs. Beall or yourself?
   - Based on this practice, what changes will you make when you ambulate someone who is weak and unsteady in a clinical setting?

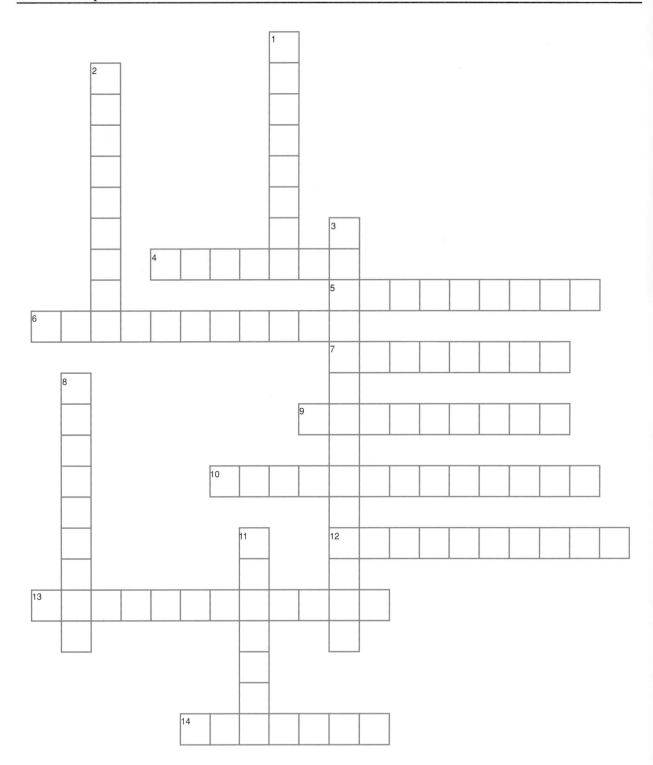

ACROSS

4. Decrease in size or a wasting away of tissue
5. Turning downward
6. Lack of joint mobility caused by abnormal shortening of a muscle
7. Turning the joint
9. Straightening of a body part
10. Movement of a joint to the extent possible without causing pain (3 words)
12. Turning upward
13. Bending the toes and foot up at the ankles
14. Brief loss of consciousness; fainting

DOWN

1. Foot falls down at the ankle (permanent plantar flexion)
2. Moving a body part toward the midline of the body
3. Excessive straightening of a body part
8. Moving a body part away from the midline of the body
11. Bending a body part

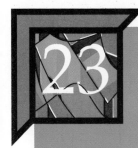

Home Management

Matching

Match the symbol with the correct instructions.

1. _____ Do not iron or press.
     a. \ 50°

2. _____ Hang to dry after removing excess water.
     b. ▢

3. _____ Use chlorine bleach with care.
     c. ◯

4. _____ Machine wash in warm water at a normal setting.
     d. △

5. _____ Hand wash gently in cool water.
     e. ⊠

6. _____ Dry clean.
     f. 🖐

True or False

*Circle **T** for true or **F** for false. Rewrite all of the false statements to make them true.*

7. **T F** Work from dirtiest to cleanest.

_____

_____

8. **T F** Dust from higher surfaces to lower surfaces.

_____

_____

9. **T F** Use plastic gloves when cleaning.

_____

_____

10. **T F** It is safe to use any cleaner in the bathroom.

_____

_____

11. **T F** A client recovering from surgery may need extra cleaning done in the bathroom.

_____

_____

12. **T F** Baking soda will remove stains.

_____

_____

13. **T F**   Any type of soap can be used in the dish-washer.

_____

_____

14. **T F**   Sort clothing by colours before washing.

_____

_____

15. **T F**   Stained items should be soaked in bleach for 10 minutes before washing.

_____

_____

16. **T F**   It is better to dry clothes in a dryer than to hang them outside.

_____

_____

17. **T F**   It is safe to mix chlorine bleach and ammonia to make a stronger cleaner.

_____

_____

Fill-In-the-Blanks

18. In order to complete home management tasks, you need to use your time wisely. Some points that will help you are

a. _____

b. _____

c. _____

d. _____

e. _____

f. _____

19. To remove urine stains, you should

a. _____

b. _____

c. _____

d. _____

e. _____

20. Your goal when doing laundry is

_____

_____

_____

21. When cleaning kitchens, you should remember

a. _____

b. _____

c. _____

d. _____

e. _____

f. _____

g. _____

22. What can you do to decrease microbes in the bathroom?

a. _____

b. _____

c. _____

d. _____

e. _____

23. Cleaning products can cause harm if not used properly. Remember to

   a. _____

   b. _____

   c. _____

   d. _____

   e. _____

   f. _____

24. What are some general cleaning guidelines?

   a. _____

   b. _____

   c. _____

   d. _____

   e. _____

   f. _____

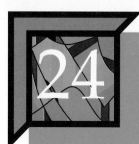

Beds and Bedmaking

Fill-In-the-Blanks

1. Describe each of the following:

   a. Closed bed

   _____

   b. Open bed

   _____

   c. Occupied bed

   _____

   d. Surgical bed

   _____

2. Why is a plastic drawsheet used on the bed?

   _____

3 What is the disadvantage of using a plastic drawsheet?

   _____

4. Why should you never shake the bed linens?

   _____

5. When making an occupied bed, the person should be covered with a bath blanket to provide

   _____ and

   _____.

6. When you are making an occupied bed, what concerns should you have about the person in the bed?

   a. _____

   b. _____

   c. _____

7. Why should you make as much of one side of the bed as possible before going to the other side?

   _____

8. What are the safety rules about using bumper pads on a crib?

   a. _____

   b. _____

   c. _____

   d. _____

9. What are the five basic bed positions?

   a. _____

   b. _____

   c. _____

   d. _____

   e. _____

Linen Scramble

10. You are getting ready to change bed linens. Number the linens you collect in the correct order from 1 to 13.

   _____ Bedspread   _____ Washcloth

   _____ Plastic drawsheet   _____ Mattress pad

   _____ Bath towel   _____ Top sheet

   _____ Bottom sheet   _____ Pillowcases

   _____ Bath blanket   _____ Blanket

   _____ Cotton drawsheet   _____ Hand towel

   _____ Hospital gown

True or False

Circle **T** *for true or* **F** *for false. Rewrite all false statements to make them true.*

11. **T** **F** In long-term care, an open bed is made because most of the residents are out of bed all day.

   _____

   _____

12. **T** **F** Residents in nursing centers may use their own linens.

   _____

   _____

13. **T** **F** If a person in home care refuses to have linens changed, you should allow the person to decide and not change the linens.

   _____

   _____

14. **T** **F** The space between the mattress and crib sides should be no more than 5 cm.

   _____

   _____

15. **T** **F** A surgical bed is made by fanfolding the linens to the side of the bed closest to the door.

   _____

   _____

Circle the Correct Answer

16. When you are changing bed linens, when should you wear gloves?
   a. At all times
   b. When linens are soiled with blood, body fluids, or body secretions or excretions
   c. When you are handling the clean linens
   d. Before the person has had a bath

17. Which statement is true when you are making an occupied bed?
   a. The person gets up and sits in a chair while you make the bed
   b. You must keep the person in good alignment while making the bed
   c. The top linens are folded so that a person can be transferred from a stretcher to the bed easily
   d. The occupied bed is made after a person is discharged from the facility

18. Why do you raise the level of the bed when you are changing linens?
   a. So that you can use good body mechanics to prevent injury
   b. To prevent injury to the person in bed
   c. To allow space under the bed for cleaning
   d. So that you can keep the person in good body alignment

Labelling

19. Name each piece of linen on bed.

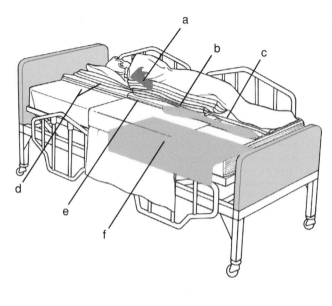

a. _____

b. _____

c. _____

d. _____

e. _____

f. _____

20. Arrange in order the steps used to make a mitred corner.

_____

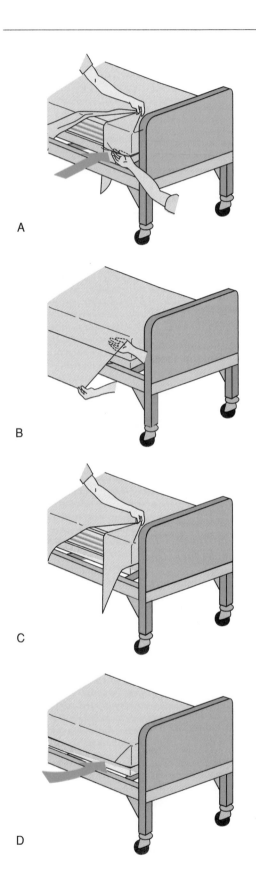

A

B

C

D

Independent Learning Activities

1. When you make beds this week, follow the new methods you have learned. Use these statements as a guide. How did these new techniques change your bedmaking practices? How many steps did you save by being organized?
   - Gather linens in the order they will be used.
   - Remove old linens and carry without touching them to your body.
   - Make as much of one side of the bed as you can before moving to the opposite side.
   - Make mitred corners when possible.
   - Place pillows with opening facing away from the doorway.

2. Role-play making an occupied bed with a classmate. Take turns playing the role of the person in the bed and the support worker. Answer the questions about the experience.

   SITUATION: Mr. Myers is 87 years old with arthritis. He has severe joint pain and is on complete bedrest at present. You plan to change his bed after completing his bath. He can turn fairly well, but you must be careful to keep his legs in good alignment with a firm pillow between the legs.
   - How did you determine what linens you needed? In what order did you gather the linens?
   - What did you tell Mr. Myers about the procedure? How did you provide for his privacy?
   - What was your first step? How did you position Mr. Myers? How did you provide for his safety?
   - How well were you able to keep the dirty and clean linens separated?
   - What difficulties did you have in following the correct procedure?
   - What changes will you make the next time you make an occupied bed?
   - What suggestions did your classmate have for you to make it more comfortable for the person in the bed?

3. Make a list in a small notebook or on an index card of the correct order of gathering linens. Carry this with you when you are in the clinical area to help you remember to be organized. Soon you will be able to gather the linens without a reminder.

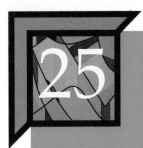

Basic Nutrition and Fluids

Fill-In-the-Blanks

1. Convert the following amounts into cubic centimetres (cc) or milliliters (mL) using this scale.
   1 oz = 30 cc (mL)
   1 cup = 240 cc (mL)
   1 quart = 1000 cc (mL)

   a. 6 oz cup of coffee =

   $6 \times 30 = 180\ cc$

   b. 8 oz of milk =

   $8 \times 30 = 240\ cc$

   c. 1 quart of water =

   $1 \times 1000 = 1000\ cc$

   d. 2 cups of tea =

   $2 \times 240 = 480\ cc$

   e. 4 oz of gelatin =

   $4 \times 30 = 120\ cc$

   f. 5 oz of orange juice =

   $5 \times 30 = 150\ cc$

   g. 12 oz of broth =

   $12 \times 30 = 360\ cc$

   h. 1/2 cup of sherbet =

   $1/2 \times 240 = 120\ cc$

2. How many calories are in

   a. 1 g of carbohydrate?

   4 calories

   b. 1 g of fat?

   9 calories

   c. 1 g of protein?

   4 calories

3. Chopped foods may be added to an infant's diet at

   about _____ of age.

4. What dietary guidelines are recommended for healthy eating?

   a. _____

   b. _____

   c. _____

   d. _____

   e. _____

5. How large is one serving of meat, poultry, or fish?

_____

How many servings of meat, poultry, or fish are recommended daily?

_____

6. In what country is beef generally not eaten?

_____

7. What would be the best way you could help to prepare these people to eat?

a. Person who must stay in bed

_____

b. Person who is allowed up out of bed

_____

8. In what ways, other than positioning, can you assist a person to get ready for meals?

a. _____

b. _____

c. _____

d. _____

e. _____

f. _____

9. How do these physical changes affect the older person's appetite or food intake?

a. Decrease in saliva

_____

b. Taste and smell dull

_____

c. Secretion of digestive juices decreases

_____

d. Loss of teeth and ill-fitting dentures

_____

e. Decreased peristalsis

_____

10. If an older person must avoid high-fibre foods, what foods may be eaten to prevent constipation?

_____

11. Why are the following actions important for safety and comfort when feeding a person?

a. Provide a relaxed mood

_____

b. Provide time and privacy to pray

_____

c. Use spoon to feed

_____

d. Offer small portions (spoon that is $1/3$ tsp full)

_____

e. Offer fluids during meal

_____

f. Engage in conversation

_____

g. Sit so you face person

_____

h. Encourage to feed him/herself

_____

12. What type of special diet would be ordered for the following situations?

   a. First diet after surgery

   _____

   b. Constipation and colon disorders

   _____

   c. Weight gain and certain thyroid imbalances

   _____

   d. Heart disease, gallbladder disease

   _____

   e. Burns, high fever, infection

   _____

13. If there is too much sodium in the diet, the body

   retains more _____.

   This increases the workload on the

   _____.

14. On a sodium-restricted diet, what is the only food group that has no restrictions?

   _____

15. The person with diabetes must eat at regular times

   to maintain _____

   _____.

16. When a person has dysphagia, what is done to the food to meet the person's needs?

   _____

17. What are six common causes of dehydration?

   a. _____

   b. _____

   c. _____

   d. _____

   e. _____

   f. _____

18. How much water does an adult need each day to survive?

   _____

19. How much fluid is needed each day to maintain normal fluid balance?

   _____

20. When fluids are restricted, why is frequent oral hygiene important?

   _____

21. List the four food groups included in the Food Guide and the number of servings for each.

   a. _____

   b. _____

   c. _____

   d. _____

22. Identify the food group to which each of the following items belong.

    a. Crackers _____

    b. Kidney beans _____

    c. Potatoes _____

    d. Pineapple chunks _____

    e. Peanut butter _____

    f. Ice milk _____

    g. Candy bar _____

    h. Oatmeal _____

    i. Carrots _____

    j. Sour cream _____

23. Should an older person increase or decrease these dietary elements? Why or when?

    a. Calories _____

       Why? _____

    b. Fluids _____

       Why? _____

    c. Protein _____

       Why? _____

    d. Soft bulk _____

       Why? _____

    e. Fried, fatty foods _____

       Why? _____

Circle the Correct Answer

24. Why are carbohydrates important in the diet?
    a. Supply products for tissue growth and repair
    b. Provide energy and bulk for bowel elimination
    c. Provide energy and flavour
    d. Supply vitamins that are needed daily

25. What can you give a person who has an order for NPO?
    a. Unlimited fluids
    b. No food or fluids
    c. Small amounts of fluids
    d. Only clear liquids

26. What effect may cultural and religious beliefs have on nutrition?
    a. Certain types of food may be restricted
    b. Method of preparation may be part of beliefs
    c. Certain foods are eaten and others are avoided
    d. All of the above may be part of beliefs

27. Which of these foods would *not* be included as liquid intake?
    a. Tomato soup
    b. Cream of wheat cereal
    c. Beef vegetable soup
    d. Chocolate pudding

28. Which of the following statements describes assistive dining?
    a. One person is fed by one support worker to reduce stimulation.
    b. Food is placed on platters or dishes and the people serve themselves.
    c. People are served food at the table as in a restaurant.
    d. Four persons are seated at the horseshoe-shaped table and are fed by one support worker.

True or False

Circle **T** *for true or* **F** *for false. Rewrite all false statements to make them true.*

29. **T   F**   The body becomes swollen if too much sugar is retained.

_____

_____

30. **T   F**   When a healthy person eats more sodium than the body needs, it will be excreted.

_____

_____

31. **T   F**   A person with diabetes will retain salt in the body.

_____

_____

32. **T   F**   A "moderate sodium-restricted diet" allows the person to eat pickles and olives.

_____

_____

33. **T   F**   When a person has diabetes, sugar builds up in the bloodstream.

_____

_____

34. **T   F**   When a person is placed on a diabetic diet, only three meals each day are allowed.

_____

_____

35. **T   F**   A diet that allows water, gelatin, and popsicles would be a clear liquid diet.

_____

_____

36. **T   F**   A person who has constipation may be helped by a high-fibre diet.

_____

_____

37. **T   F**   Many special diets involve between-meal nourishments such as crackers and milk.

_____

_____

Matching

Match the nutrient with the reason it is important to good health.

38. _____   Needed for tooth and bone formation   a. Protein

39. _____   Tissue growth and repair   b. Carbohydrates

40. _____   Provides energy and adds flavour   c. Fats

41. _____   Provides energy and fibre for elimination   d. Vitamins

42. _____   Does not provide calories, but needed for certain body functions   e. Minerals

Match the vitamin with its major function.

43. _____ Healthy eyes, healthy skin and mucous membranes, protein and carbo-hydrate metabolism

44. _____ Formation of substances that hold tissues together

45. _____ Formation of red blood cells, nervous system functioning

46. _____ Blood clotting

47. _____ Normal reproduction

48. _____ Growth, vision, healthy hair, and skin

49. _____ Muscle tone, nerve function, digestion

50. _____ Protein, fat, and carbohydrate metabolism

51. _____ Formation of red blood cells, functioning of intestine

52. _____ Absorption and metabolism of calcium and phosphorus, healthy bones

a. Vitamin A

b. Thiamine

c. Riboflavin

d. Niacin

e. Vitamin B12

f. Folic acid

g. Ascorbic acid

h. Vitamin D

i. Vitamin E

j. Vitamin K

Match the mineral with its major function.

53. _____ Formation of bone and teeth, nerve and muscle function

54. _____ Thyroid gland function

55. _____ Fluid balance

56. _____ Formation of bone, teeth, blood clotting

57. _____ Allows red blood cells to carry oxygen

58. _____ Nerve function, heart function

a. Calcium

b. Phosphorus

c. Iron

d. Iodine

e. Sodium

f. Potassium

Labelling

59. Label the plate with numbers so that you could de-scribe the location of food to a blind person.
    a. Where would you tell the blind person to find the meat?

    _____

    b. Where would you tell the blind person to find the baked potato?

    _____

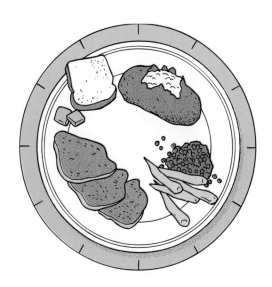

Independent Learning Activities

1. How well balanced is your diet? Make a list of all of the foods and fluids you eat and drink for 1 day. Jot down the list as soon as you eat so that you do not forget anything. Make sure that you estimate the amount of each food you eat. Remember that size is important when counting servings! Organize the list. Answer these questions about your diet.
    * How many servings did you eat of breads, cereals, rice, and pasta? How many of these servings were whole-grain products?
    * How many fruit servings did you eat? Were these servings fresh or canned?
    * How many vegetable servings did you eat? Were the vegetables raw or cooked?
    * How many servings of milk, yogurt, and cheese were in your diet? Were these products low-fat?
    * How many servings of meat, fish, dry beans, eggs, and nuts did you have? Were the choices you made high in fat or salt?
    * How many foods did you eat that only count as fats, oils, or sweets?
    * In which groups are you meeting the daily needs?
    * In which groups are you eating more than is needed for a healthy diet?
    * In which groups do you need to increase your intake to have a healthy diet?
    * How did this exercise help you to consider changes in your eating habits so that your diet will be healthier?

2. With a classmate, role-play feeding a person. Take turns as the person being fed. You may choose any spoon-fed foods you wish. (Pudding, gelatin, and soup are suggestions.) You should also have a beverage to give the person.

    Consider these questions and discuss how you felt when you were the person being fed.
    * How were your physical needs (elimination, oral care, handwashing) met before the meal started?
    * Where were you fed (bed, chair)? Who made the decision about your location?
    * Which food was offered first? Who made the choice? How was the food offered? All of one type until it was gone? A variety throughout the meal? Were you asked what you preferred?
    * When was a beverage offered? Was it as hot or cold as you preferred? Were you given a choice about the temperature?
    * How was the person feeding you positioned? Did the person's posture make you feel comfortable? Rushed?
    * What opportunities were offered to talk or rest during the meal? Did you feel relaxed or rushed?
    * After this exercise, what will you do differently when you feed a person?

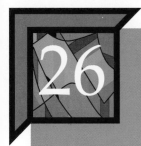

26

Enteral Nutrition and IV Therapy

True or False

Circle **T** *for true or* **F** *for false. Rewrite all false statements to make them true.*

1. **T F**   During a scheduled tube feeding, 400 mL is usually given over 20 minutes.

   _____

   _____

2. **T F**   Formula for feeding tubes should be heated.

   _____

   _____

3. **T F**   Risk of regurgitation is less with nasointestinal tubes.

   _____

   _____

4. **T F**   Mouth care is not important when clients are NPO.

   _____

   _____

5. **T F**   An IV site on the back of the hand is in a central venous site.

   _____

   _____

Circle the Correct Answer

6. Which of the following describes a gastrostomy tube?
   a. A tube is inserted through a surgical opening into the stomach.
   b. A tube is inserted through the nose into the stomach.
   c. An opening is made into the middle part of the small intestine.
   d. A tube is inserted through the nose into the duodenum.

7. What responsibility does the support worker have if a person is being fed through a tube?
   a. Remove the tube after each feeding
   b. Give clear liquids by mouth
   c. Assist the nurse in giving feedings
   d. Avoid giving mouth care

8. People who cannot chew or swallow often receive nutrition by
   a. Enteral nutrition
   b. IV feedings
   c. A liquid diet
   d. A puréed diet

9. What should be reported to the RN about the flow rate when the person has an IV?
   a. No fluid is dripping
   b. The rate is too fast
   c. The rate is too slow
   d. All of the above

Fill-In-the-Blanks

10. Feeding tubes are inserted into the GI tract through different routes. List the routes and briefly describe each one.

   a. _____

   _____

   b. _____

   _____

   c. _____

   _____

   d. _____

   _____

   e. _____

   _____

11. What conditions may require a client to have a feeding tube?

   a. _____

   b. _____

   c. _____

   d. _____

   e. _____

12. What can cause the feeding tube to move?

   a. _____

   b. _____

   c. _____

   d. _____

   e. _____

13. When you care for a client at home with a feeding tube, you should never

   a. _____

   b. _____

   c. _____

14. Scheduled enteral feedings are usually given _____ a day. About _____ mL are given over _____ minutes.

15. Continuous enteral feedings require an _____.

16. When a person is receiving an enteral feeding, he/she sits or is in a _____ position for at least _____ after the feeding. This position helps to prevent _____.

17. How do these measures help the person with a feeding tube feel more comfortable?

   a. Hard candy or gum

   _____

   b. Lubricant for lips

   _____

   c. Cleaning of nose and nostrils every 4 to 8 hours

   _____

   d. Frequent oral hygiene

   _____

18. Why is the left side-lying position avoided when a person is receiving enteral nutrition?

   _____

19. What should be reported to the nurse if the person is receiving a tube feeding?

   a. _____

   b. _____

   c. _____

   d. _____

   e. _____

f. _____

g. _____

h. _____

i. _____

j. _____

k. _____

l. _____

20. A person may receive IV therapy to

a. _____

b. _____

c. _____

d. _____

e. _____

21. You may care for people who have IVs in different sites. Explain where each of these IVs would be inserted.

a. Peripheral

_____

b. Scalp

_____

c. Central venous sites

_____

d. Peripherally inserted central catheter (PICC)

_____

22. What safety measures must be followed when the person has an IV?

a. _____

b. _____

c. _____

d. _____

e. _____

f. _____

g. _____

h. _____

23. What are the signs and symptoms that indicate there is a problem with an IV site?

At the IV site:

a. _____

b. _____

c. _____

d. _____

e. _____

Systemic signs and symptoms:

f. _____

g. _____

h. _____

i. _____

j. _____

k. _____

l. _____

m. _____

n. _____

o. _____

p. _____

q. _____

r. _____

s. _____

Personal Hygiene

Matching

Match the following statements with the time the care described is usually given. Some of the descriptions will have more than one answer. List all correct answers.

1. _____ Shaving person

2. _____ Giving back massage

3. _____ Helping person to undress and put on pyjamas

4. _____ Taking to the bathroom or offering bedpan or urinal

5. _____ Brushing or combing the person's hair

6. _____ Straightening unit

a. AM care

b. Morning care

c. Afternoon care

d. HS care

Fill-In-the-Blanks

7. When should oral hygiene be offered?

   a. _____

   b. _____

   c. _____

   d. _____

8. What causes these problems in the oral cavity?

   a. Bad taste

   _____

   b. White coating on tongue

   _____

c. Redness and swelling of tongue and mouth

_____

d. Dry mouth

_____

9. Children should learn to brush their teeth at about

   age _____.

10. When giving oral care, what observations should you report to the nurse?

   a. _____

   b. _____

   c. _____

   d. _____

   e. _____

   f. _____

11. When you are cleaning dentures, why do you fill the sink or basin with water and line it with a towel?

   _____

12. Hot water should not be used to clean or store dentures because it may cause them to

   _____

13. Why should dentures be stored in water?

   _____

14. What are the reasons the teeth should be flossed?

   a. _____

   b. _____

15. When giving mouth care to an unconscious person, it is important to turn the person

   _____

   to prevent _____.

16. What are reasons for bathing a person?

   a. _____

   b. _____

   c. _____

   d. _____

17. If an older person with dementia resists your effort to assist with hygiene, you may find ways to work with the person in the

   _____.

18. Why are older people with dementia sometimes agitated and combative during bathing procedures?

   a. _____

   b. _____

19. How can the support worker help the person with dementia to tolerate a bath?

   a. _____

   b. _____

   c. _____

   d. _____

20. Why are the following rules important when bathing a person?

   a. Keep soap in dish between lathering

   _____

   b. Rinse the skin

   _____

   c. Pat the skin dry

   _____

   d. Bathe the skin whenever urine and feces are present

   _____

21. How can you provide for warmth during a bath?

    a. _____

    b. _____

22. Where is powder generally applied?

    _____

23. What can happen when too much powder is used?

    _____

24. Lower water temperature for bathing is important

    for _____ because

    they have _____ .

25. When giving a tub bath or shower, what safety measures will help to prevent falls?

    a. _____

    b. _____

    c. _____

    d. _____

    e. _____

    f. _____

    g. _____

    h. _____

    i. _____

    j. _____

26. What observations should you make and report when you give a person a bath?

    a. _____

    b. _____

    c. _____

    d. _____

e. _____

f. _____

g. _____

h. _____

27. What areas are bathed when giving a partial bath?

    a. _____

    b. _____

    c. _____

    d. _____

    e. _____

    f. _____

28. The tub or shower should be cleaned before using

    to prevent _____ .

29. What are four reasons a complete bed bath may be ordered?

    a. _____

    b. _____

    c. _____

    d. _____

30. Why is the water temperature for a bed bath 43.3° to 46.1° C?

    _____

31. When washing and drying the chest during a bed bath, what steps are taken to avoid exposing the person?

    a. _____

    b. _____

    c. _____

32. Back massages should not be given to people with:

    a. _____

    b. _____

    c. _____

    d. _____

    e. _____

33. The cleanest area in the perineal area is the

    _____ and the dirtiest

    area is the _____.

34. When giving perineal care, what observations should be reported to the nurse?

    a. _____

    b. _____

    c. _____

Circle the Correct Answer

35. When giving oral care, why should you wear gloves?
    a. You will have contact with the mucous membranes.
    b. The gums may bleed.
    c. There may be harmful bacteria (pathogens) in the mouth.
    d. All of the above are correct.

36. Mouth care should be given to an unconscious person
    a. once a day.
    b. once each shift.
    c. after every meal.
    d. every 2 hours.

37. You should avoid using bath oils when giving a tub bath or shower because they
    a. make the tub or floor slippery.
    b. may be irritating to the skin.
    c. will cause dryness of the skin.
    d. may collect in skin folds and cause skin breakdown.

38. Before being given a bath, the person should be assisted to the bathroom or offered the commode, bedpan, or urinal because
    a. this will prevent incontinence during the bath.
    b. bathing stimulates urination.
    c. it will prevent skin breakdown during the bath.
    d. it will prevent soiling after the bath.

39. When giving a back massage, it should last about
    a. 1 to 2 minutes.
    b. 3 to 5 minutes.
    c. 6 to 8 minutes.
    d. at least 10 minutes.

40. What is one reason to provide perineal care at least once a day?
    a. To prevent the growth of microbes that cause infection
    b. To prevent incontinence
    c. To prevent pain
    d. To provide exercise

41. Which of the following is the correct way to wash the perineal area?
    a. Wash from the anal area toward the urethra
    b. Wash in a circular motion from the outside to the inside
    c. Wash from the urethra to the anal area
    d. Wash back and forth over the entire area several times

42. The bath water is changed during a complete bed bath
    a. after washing the chest and abdomen if the water is soapy or cool.
    b. before washing the feet and legs.
    c. after giving perineal care.
    d. only if it is soapy or cool.

43. Which of these steps is not correct when giving male perineal care?
    a. Retract the foreskin of the uncircumcised male
    b. Wash the tip of the penis starting at the urethral opening and working outward
    c. Clean the shaft of the penis with firm, downward strokes
    d. Leave the foreskin retracted at the end of the procedure

True or False

Circle **T** *for true or* **F** *for false. Rewrite all false statements to make them true.*

44. **T   F**   Soap dries the skin, especially in older persons.

_____

_____

45. **T   F**   The support worker decides what skin care products to use when giving a bath.

_____

_____

46. **T   F**   Plain water may be used for the bath when the skin is very dry.

_____

_____

47. **T   F**   Bath oils and lotions are used to clean the skin.

_____

_____

48. **T   F**   Adjust the water temperature and pressure before the person gets in the shower.

_____

_____

Labelling

49. Using arrows, show the directions in which the teeth should be brushed.

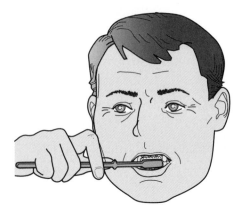

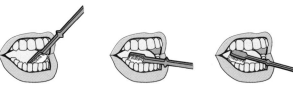

50. Using an arrow, show the direction used to clean the eyes while giving a bedbath.

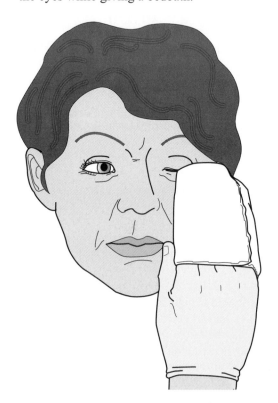

51. Draw lines with arrows to show the direction your
    hands move when giving a backrub.

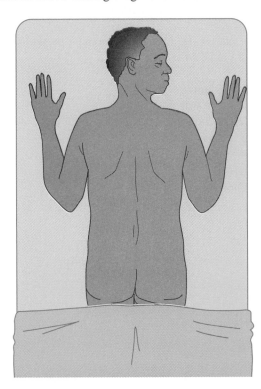

Independent Learning Activities

1. Have three or four classmates answer these questions to discover differences in personal hygiene practices.
   How does this comparison help you to understand differences in personal hygiene practices of your patients or
   residents?
   • How often do you usually take a complete bath or shower?
   • Do you prefer a shower or a tub bath?
   • What time of day do you usually bathe?
   • What methods do you use to keep skin healthy? Special soaps? Lotions? Bath oils?
   • When do you prefer to brush your teeth? How many times a day do you brush? How often do you floss?
     What type of brush and toothpaste do you prefer?
   • What type of deodorant or antiperspirant do you use? Roll-on? Spray?

2. Role-play this situation with a classmate. Take turns as the support worker and the person receiving the back
   rub.

   SITUATION: You are assigned to give Mrs. Leland a back rub at bedtime. You know that she is confused and
   cannot communicate with you, so you cannot ask her how she likes to have her back rub done. You try a variety of strokes and techniques in an effort to make Mrs. Leland comfortable.

   Consider these questions about how you felt when you were "Mrs. Leland."
   • How did the lotion feel on your back? Was it warm or cold?
   • Which strokes were more relaxing? More stimulating? Which did you prefer?
   • How long do you think that the back rub lasted? How did you know that the back rub was ending? What
     nonverbal clues did you sense?
   • What would you like to tell the person giving the back rub that would improve the technique used?

3. Using the directions in your textbook, make a padded tongue blade that could be used when giving oral hygiene. What is the purpose of the padded tongue blade?
4. Role-play this situation with a classmate. Take turns as the support worker and the person receiving oral care.

SITUATION: Mr. Adams, 78, fractured his right shoulder in a fall. He has left-sided weakness from a stroke (CVA, brain attack). You are assigned to provide oral hygiene, including flossing.

Consider these questions about how you felt when you were "Mr. Adams."
- What did the support worker explain to you before the oral hygiene was done?
- What choices were you given? About positioning or equipment? About products used? About techniques used?
- How did it feel to have someone else give you oral care? Flossing your teeth?
- How clean did your teeth feel when the oral care was completed?
- What would you like to tell the person giving the oral care about the techniques used?

28

Grooming and Dressing

Fill-In-the-Blanks

1. Brushing and combing are important to prevent

_____ in long hair.

2. What specific measures are needed for curly, coarse, dry hair?

   a. _____

   b. _____

   c. _____

3. What can you do to maintain safety and comfort with different methods of shampooing?

   a. During shower or bath

   _____

   b. At sink

   _____

   c. On stretcher

   _____

   d. In bed

   _____

4. What should you do if the person asks to have his/her hair washed?

   _____

5. Shampooing at the sink or on a stretcher is difficult

   for _____.

6. Why should you follow Standard Precautions when shaving a person?

   _____

7. An adolescent may need frequent shampooing be-

   cause _____.

8. When making a plastic trough to wash hair in the bed at home, you should not use

   _____.

9. How can you soften the skin before shaving?

   _____

10. If nicks or cuts occur when shaving a person, you should

a. _____

b. _____

11. When you are giving foot care, what is one thing you must not do?

_____

12. How do the following factors help to cause foot injury, infection, or odours?

a. Dirty feet, socks, stockings

_____

b. Shoes and socks

_____

c. Poorly fitted shoes

_____

d. Poor circulation

_____

e. Diabetes, vascular diseases

_____

f. Trimming/cutting toenails

_____

13. _____ and

_____ are

serious complications of foot injuries.

14. When is the best time to clean and trim fingernails?

_____

15. List four observations are reported to the nurse when observed during foot care?

a. _____

b. _____

c. _____

d. _____

16. Number the following steps in the correct order for undressing a person.

_____ Remove pullover garments
_____ Remove garments that open in the front
_____ Cover the person with a bath blanket
_____ Undo buttons, zippers, or ties on garments that open in the front
_____ Remove pants or slacks
_____ Remove garments that open in the back

Circle the Correct Answer

17. A person has long hair. Which procedure cannot be done?
a. Daily brushing and combing
b. Shampooing
c. Cutting the hair to remove tangles and matting
d. Braiding or styling

18. A woman in a long-term care facility has her hair done weekly at the beauty shop. During her shower you should
a. wash her hair as usual.
b. protect her hair with a shower cap.
c. be careful not to get water on her hair during the shower.
d. wrap a towel around her head to protect her hair.

19. Which of these should you wear when you are shaving a person?
a. Gown
b. Gloves
c. Mask
d. Gown, gloves, and mask

20. Which of these statements is correct about dressing or undressing a person?
    a. Remove clothing from the weak side first
    b. Put clothing on the weak side first
    c. Put clothing on the strong side first
    d. Remove clothing from the side farthest away from you first

21. Which of these steps is correct when you change a gown for a person with an IV?
    a. Remove the gown from the arm with the IV first
    b. Gather up the sleeve of the arm with the IV and slide it over the IV site and tubing
    c. Turn off the IV and disconnect it temporarily while changing the gown
    d. Put the gown on the arm without the IV first

Matching

Match the words related to personal care with the descriptions below.

22. _____ Excessive body hair

23. _____ Infestation with lice in the pubic area

24. _____ Hair loss

25. _____ An infestation with lice

26. _____ You may groom hair in this manner with the person's permission

27. _____ Excessive amounts of dry, white flakes from the scalp

28. _____ Parasites that can live on different parts of the body

29. _____ You must never do this to matted or tangled hair

30. _____ Infestation of the scalp with lice

31. _____ Infestation of the body with lice

a. Cutting

b. Pediculosis pubis

c. Hirsutism

d. Pediculosis capitis

e. Dandruff

f. Pediculosis

g. Alopecia

h. Pediculosis corporis

i. Lice

j. Braiding

True or False

Circle **T** *for true or* **F** *for false. Rewrite all false statements to make them true.*

32. **T** **F** How the hair looks has no effect on the person's well-being.

_____

_____

33. **T** **F** When brushing hair, start at the scalp and brush to the hair ends.

_____

_____

34. **T** **F** If hair is tangled and matted, first start to brush at the scalp and brush to the ends.

_____

_____

35. **T** **F** When caring for adolescents, style hair in a manner that pleases the child and parents.

_____

_____

36. **T** **F** Older people need to shampoo more frequently because of decreased oil gland secretion.

_____

_____

37. **T** **F** A woman may want you to shave coarse facial hair.

_____

_____

38. **T** **F** When shaving the face, the skin should be loose.

_____

_____

39. **T** **F** Fingernails should be trimmed with scissors.

_____

_____

Independent Learning Activities

1. Think about how you shave a part of your body (legs, face, underarms, and so on) and answer the following questions that apply.
    *   What type of equipment works best? New or used blade or razor? Safety razor or disposable razor?
    *   What difference does it make if you use shaving cream? Soapy lather? Water alone?
    *   What happens if you try to shave without any lubricant such as shaving cream? How does the skin feel? How does the razor move across the skin? What problem(s) may occur if this method is used?
    *   Which technique makes shaving easier? When you apply more pressure? Less pressure? Shaving against the hair growth? With the hair growth?
    *   Shave one leg or one side of the face with the hair growth and the other leg or side of the face against the hair growth. What difference in the hair growth can you notice in the next day or two?
    *   What areas are most difficult to shave? How do you deal with these areas?

2. Role play this situation with a classmate with each of you taking turns as the person being dressed and the support worker. When you are acting as Mr. Olson, remember to keep your left arm and leg limp. Answer the questions about dressing a person.

    SITUATION: Mr. Olson is an 58 year old who has weakness on the left side of his body. You are assigned to help him dress in regular clothes after breakfast. He is sitting in a chair in his room wearing pyjamas, a robe, and slippers. His fresh clothes are on the bed, including an undershirt, dress shirt, slacks, socks, and shoes.
    *   How did you provide for Mr. Olson's privacy?
    *   How did you position Mr. Olson to undress and dress him?
    *   How did you remove his robe? Pyjamas? Slippers?
    *   How did you get an over-the-head undershirt on Mr. Olson?
    *   Which arm did you redress first? Was this effective or did you have difficulty?
    *   What difficulties did you have getting the dress shirt on Mr. Olson?
    *   How did you put on the slacks? What difficulties did you have with this?
    *   How did you put on the socks and shoes?
    *   Overall, was this procedure easier or harder than you thought it would be? Were you able to follow the directions in Chapter 28 of the textbook to make this task easier?
    *   Discuss with each other how you felt when you were Mr. Olson and you were unable to assist in getting dressed.

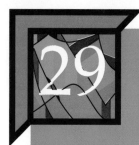

Urinary Elimination

Fill-In-the-Blanks

1. How much urine does an adult normally produce every day?

   _____

2. When do most people usually void during the day? (Normal voiding routine)

   a. _____

   b. _____

   c. _____

3. What effects do each of these have on urine?

   a. Coffee, tea, alcohol

   _____

   b. Diet high in salt

   _____

   c. Beets, blackberries

   _____

   d. Carrots, sweet potatoes

   _____

   e. Asparagus

   _____

4. When may a fracture (bed)pan be used?

   a. _____

   b. _____

   c. _____

   d. _____

5. Why does a urinal have a hooked handle?

   _____

6. If a person is embarrassed about voiding with others close by, what can be done to mask the sounds?

   _____

7. When you leave a person alone to void you should

   place the _____ and

   _____ within reach.

8. How can you promote relaxation and not rush the person who is voiding?

   a. _____

   b. _____

9. After a person has voided, you should provide

   _____

   care as needed and have the person

   _____ .

10. Why should you wear gloves when emptying a bedpan or urinal?

    _____

11. If a urinary drainage bag is higher than the bladder,

    urine can _____ and an

    _____ can develop.

12. Why must you *never* use adhesive tape to secure a condom catheter?

    _____

13. When securing a condom catheter in place, how is tape applied?

    _____

14. What measures can you take to help people with urinary incontinence?

    a. _____

    b. _____

    c. _____

    d. _____

    e. _____

    f. _____

    g. _____

    h. _____

    i. _____

    j. _____

15. What disorders and other conditions may cause urinary incontinence?

    a. Disorders

       _____

    b. Other causes

       _____

16. What complications can occur when a person has incontinence?

    _____

17. The goal of bladder training is

    _____ .

18. Explain the two basic methods of bladder training.

    a. _____

    b. _____

19. When collecting a midstream urine specimen, you

    ask the resident to start _____

    into the toilet, bedpan, commode, or urinal. Then

    you pass the specimen container _____

    _____ .

20. In order to prevent the growth of microorganisms, how is a 24-hour urine specimen handled?

    _____

21. Why is urine strained?

    _____

The next five fill-in-the-blank exercises (questions 22 through 26) each describe a common urinary problem. Identify the problem and list the causes of each problem.

22. Painful or difficult urination is called

_____.

   a. _____

   b. _____

   c. _____

23. Blood in the urine is called

_____.

   a. _____

   b. _____

   c. _____

24. Frequent urination at night is called

_____.

   a. _____

   b. _____

   c. _____

25. Scant amount of urine, usually less than 500 mL in 24 hours, is called

_____.

   a. _____

   b. _____

   c. _____

   d. _____

   e. _____

26. Production of abnormally large amounts of urine is called

_____.

   a. _____

   b. _____

   c. _____

   d. _____

27. A ureterostomy is

_____

_____

Circle the Correct Answer

28. Why is voiding in a bedside commode easier than voiding in a bedpan?
   a. It allows a more normal position for elimination
   b. It provides more privacy
   c. It is more comfortable
   d. It allows the bladder to empty completely

29. Which of the following correctly describes catheter care?
   a. Wash the perineal area and avoid touching the catheter
   b. Clean the meatus and the catheter with an alcohol swab
   c. Clean the catheter from the meatus down the catheter about 10 cm with soap and water
   d. Clean the catheter with soap and water, starting about 10 cm below the meatus and washing toward the perineal area

30. When applying a condom catheter, you should use
   a. sterile technique.
   b. Standard Precautions.
   c. contact precautions.
   d. droplet precautions.

31. When a person is having a 24-hour urine specimen collected, what should you do with the first voiding?
   a. Discard it
   b. Send it to the lab
   c. Place it in the large container used for saving the urine
   d. Test it for sugar and ketones

32. Which of these actions would *not* be helpful in getting a person to void?
    a. Pull the curtains and close doors while the person is urinating
    b. Stand next to the bed and talk quietly to the person who is urinating
    c. Run water in the sink while the person is sitting on the toilet
    d. Stand outside the curtain or bathroom door while the person is urinating

33. When emptying a urinary drainage bag, you maintain medical asepsis by
    a. using sterile gloves.
    b. placing the measuring container on top of a paper towel.
    c. placing the measuring container on top of the overbed table to read it accurately.
    d. doing all of the above.

34. When straining urine, what should you do if you see particles in the strainer?
    a. Place the strainer in the container and send to the laboratory
    b. Show it to the nurse, then discard
    c. Send the urine and strainer to the laboratory
    d. Keep the strainer in the patient's room until the doctor arrives

35. When using a reagent strip to test urine, the support worker should
    a. send the specimen and reagent strip to the laboratory.
    b. ask the nurse to read the strip.
    c. follow the manufacturer's instructions on the container.
    d. teach the patient to read the strips.

True or False

*Circle **T** for true or **F** for false. Rewrite all false statements to make them true.*

36. **T   F**   When assisting with normal elimination, you should practise surgical asepsis and Standard Precautions.

_____

_____

37. **T   F**   Normal elimination is easier if a man can stand or a woman can sit or squat.

_____

_____

38. **T   F**   If a person has osteoporosis, painful joints from arthritis, or a hip replacement, a regular bedpan will be the most comfortable.

_____

_____

39. **T   F**   Incontinence is a common reason for seeking long-term care for a family member.

_____

_____

40. **T   F**   When collecting a specimen, you should use a sterile container.

_____

_____

41. **T   F**   A specimen container must be labeled with the person's initials, room and bed number, date, and time.

_____

_____

42. **T   F**   When you collect a urine specimen you should tell the person not to have a bowel movement or place toilet tissue in the container.

_____

_____

43. **T   F**   The specimen container and requisition slip are taken to the laboratory in a plastic cup.

_____

_____

Labelling

44. Draw an arrow to show the direction to clean the catheter. List observations you make that need to be reported to the nurse when caring for a person with an indwelling catheter.

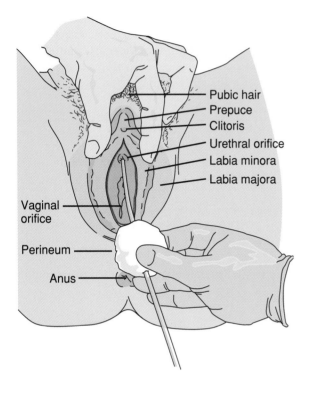

a. _____

b. _____

c. _____

d. _____

Answer questions 45 through 47 using the following illustration.

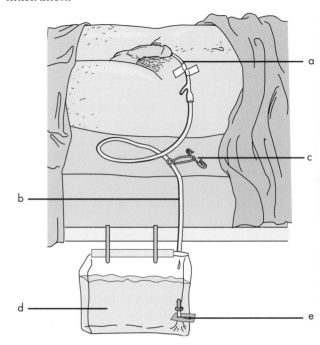

45. Name the parts of the urinary drainage system indicated.

a. _____

b. _____

c. _____

d. _____

e. _____

46. Why is the tubing coiled on the bed?

_____

_____

47. Why is the catheter taped to the man's abdomen?

_____

_____

Independent Learning Activities

1. Role-play this situation with a classmate. Take turns being the person using the bedpan and the support worker.

   SITUATION: Mrs. Donnelly is a 70 year old who must use the bedpan because she is on complete bed rest. She finds it difficult to move easily and usually cannot raise her hips to get on the bedpan. She tells you she will try to assist you as much as she can. You first attempt to have her lift her hips and when that method does not work well, you roll her onto the bedpan.

   Consider these questions about how you carried out this procedure as the support worker.
   - What did you do to provide privacy and safety for Mrs. Donnelly?
   - How did you position her to see if she could help you by lifting her hips?
   - What difficulties did you have getting the pan under her with her help?
   - How did you reposition Mrs. Donnelly to roll her on the pan?
   - What difficulties did you have rolling her onto the pan? How well was she positioned on the pan? What adjustments were needed to centre her on the bedpan?
   - What steps did you take to make sure she was comfortable? How was the head of the bed positioned?
   - What steps did you use to remove the pan? What difficulties did you have getting the pan out from under Mrs. Donnelly?
   - If the bedpan had had urine in it, how would you have prevented spilling during the procedure?
   - What suggestions did your classmate have to help you carry out this procedure better with a person in a health care setting?

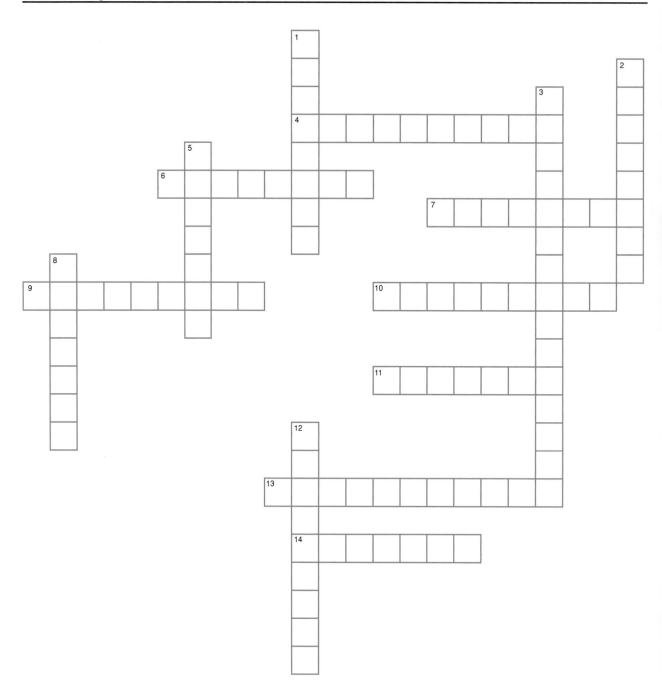

ACROSS

4. Sugar in the urine
6. Production of abnormally large amounts of urine
7. Tube used to drain or inject fluid through a body opening
9. Voiding at frequent intervals
10. Blood in the urine
11. Painful or difficult urination
13. Process of emptying urine from the bladder; urination or voiding
14. A compound that appears in the urine because of rapid breakdown of fat for energy; Ketone body.

DOWN

1. Scant amount of urine; usually less than 500 mL in 24 hours
2. Frequent urination at night
3. Process of inserting a catheter
5. Urination or micturition
8. Need to void immediately
12. Process of emptying urine from bladder; micturition or voiding

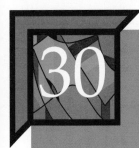

Bowel Elimination

Word Search

Write the correct word next to each definition. Find the words in the Word Search that match the definitions and circle or highlight the words.

I	B	O	W	E	L	E	L	I	M	I	N	A	T	I	O	N	S
N	S	U	N	N	Y	M	A	F	I	N	D	R	O	N	T	O	T
C	U	Q	O	L	I	T	E	E	N	L	E	A	P	F	R	O	U
O	P	U	S	T	L	C	T	N	D	A	F	S	L	L	O	L	D
N	P	A	T	G	E	N	T	L	E	M	A	K	A	A	L	A	Y
T	O	L	O	S	O	L	I	F	E	M	C	I	S	T	O	M	A
I	S	I	O	G	S	L	A	N	U	S	A	N	A	U	T	W	A
N	I	T	L	E	T	P	E	R	I	S	T	A	L	S	I	S	R
E	T	Y	O	F	O	D	R	Y	P	R	I	V	C	C	Y	M	D
N	O	S	T	O	M	Y	T	I	N	L	O	V	E	H	A	H	N
C	R	O	T	O	Y	A	K	I	N	O	N	E	S	S	Y	O	O
E	Y	L	I	F	E	D	I	A	R	R	H	E	A	S	L	M	W
B	O	W	E	L	T	R	A	I	N	I	N	G	P	L	A	N	E

1. _____ Semisolid mass of waste products in the colon

2. _____ Introduction of fluid into the rectum and lower colon

3. _____ Artificial opening between the ileum and abdomen

4. _____ Bowel movement

5. _____ Alternating contraction and relaxation of intestinal muscles

6. _____ Surgical creation of an artificial opening

7. _____ Cone-shaped medication that is inserted into a body opening

8. _____ Gas or air in the stomach or intestines

9. _____ Feces that have been excreted

10. _____ Frequent passage of liquid stools

11. _____ Partially digested food and fluids that pass from the stomach to the small intestine

12. _____ The opening of a colostomy or ileostomy

Fill-In-the-Blanks

13. What factors could cause stool to change to these colours?

   a. Black

   _____

   b. Red

   _____

   c. Green

   _____

14. What should you observe and report when a person has a bowel movement?

   a. _____

   b. _____

   c. _____

   d. _____

   e. _____

   f. _____

   g. _____

   h. _____

15. What happens to the feces when fluid intake is poor?

   _____

16. What effect does normal bacterial action in the large intestine have on the stool?

   _____

17. What are some signs of fecal impaction?

   a. _____

   b. _____

   c. _____

18. What are common causes of constipation?

   a. _____

   b. _____

   c. _____

   d. _____

   e. _____

   f. _____

   g. _____

19. What comfort and safety measures can the support worker use when assisting a person with bowel elimination?

   a. _____

   b. _____

c. _____

d. _____

e. _____

f. _____

20. What are the risks if you do not give good skin care when a person has diarrhea?

    a. _____

    b. _____

    c. _____

21. What can the support worker do that may help to prevent fecal incontinence?

    _____

22. If an infant, young child, or older person has diarrhea, it is very serious because the person would be at risk for

    _____.

23. What symptoms may occur if flatulence is not relieved?

    a. _____

    b. _____

    c. _____

24. What are two goals of bowel training?

    a. _____

    b. _____

25. When you are helping a person with bowel training, the person is usually encouraged to use the toilet, commode, or bedpan after a

    _____, usually

    _____.

26. A suppository is used to stimulate

    _____

    when bowel training is being done.

27. What are four reasons that enemas are given?

    a. _____

    b. _____

    c. _____

    d. _____

28. How would you mix the solution for a saline enema?

    _____

29. How does a commercial enema, which contains only 120 mL of solution, stimulate defecation?

    _____

30. When you are giving "enemas until clear," how will you know that you have given enough?

    _____

31. How warm is the solution in a cleansing enema?

    _____

32. Only a _____

    enema may be given to children.

33. What instructions should you give to a person who is going to expel an enema in the toilet?

    _____

34. What will happen if you release pressure on the commercial enema container?

    _____

35. What is the purpose of an ostomy pouch?

_____

36. You should empty or open an ostomy pouch when

it is _____ or when the

bag _____.

37. An ostomy bag is changed every _____ days.

38. How can odour with an ostomy pouch be prevented?

a. _____

b. _____

c. _____

d. _____

39. An ostomy pouch can be removed and changed when peristalsis is less active. The best time is usually

_____.

40. Why are the feces from an ileostomy especially irritating to the skin?

_____

41. Why are certain stool specimens taken directly to the laboratory?

_____

42. What is occult blood?

_____

Circle the Correct Answer

43. Which of the following will *not* assist bowel elimination?
    a. Drinking a hot beverage
    b. Using a bedside commode in a semiprivate room
    c. Taking a walk
    d. Reading a book or newspaper

44. Which of these foods would be more likely to stimulate bowel elimination?
    a. Pudding and gelatin
    b. Whole-grain cereals and fruit
    c. Meat and fish
    d. Pretzels and potato chips

45. Mr. Lane, 85, usually has a bowel movement after breakfast. About 45 minutes after having a bowel movement, he wants to go to the bathroom again. The most likely reason for this is
    a. older persons lose control over defecation.
    b. complete emptying of the rectum does not always occur with older persons.
    c. he may have a tumor or other disorder.
    d. he is concerned about becoming constipated.

46. Which of these may kill normal flora in the intestine?
    a. Antibiotics
    b. Laxatives
    c. Pain medications
    d. Enemas

47. What will the nurse be likely to tell you if the person has diarrhea?
    a. Withhold all fluids
    b. Give the person plenty to drink
    c. Encourage the person to eat as little as possible
    d. Give the person foods with plenty of fibre

48. What would be an effective nursing action to relieve flatulence?
    a. Give an enema
    b. Make sure the diet is high in vegetables
    c. Have the person lie flat in bed
    d. Ambulate the person or place in the side-lying position

49. When the nurse inserts a suppository to stimulate defecation, how soon would you expect results?
    a. In about 30 minutes
    b. Immediately
    c. 2 to 3 hours
    d. In the morning

50. How much solution is usually given as a cleansing enema to an adult?
    a. 500-1000 mL
    b. 400 mL
    c. 120 mL
    d. 250 mL

51. Which position is best when giving an enema?
    a. Sims' position
    b. Right position
    c. Semi-Fowler's position
    d. Prone position

52. When giving an enema, what should you do if the person complains of abdominal cramping?
    a. Insert the tube 2 cm more
    b. Clamp the tubing until the cramping stops
    c. Discontinue the enema and report it to the nurse
    d. Withdraw the tube about 2 cm

53. What is the purpose of a rectal tube?
    a. Relief of constipation
    b. Treatment of fecal impaction
    c. Prevention of diarrhea
    d. Relief of flatulence and distention

54. What is the consistency of the stool if a colostomy is near the end of the large intestine?
    a. Liquid
    b. Soft
    c. Formed
    d. Hard and dry

55. Which of these methods would help to prevent skin breakdown around the stoma?
    a. Clean with alcohol wipes
    b. Use an antiseptic lotion or petroleum jelly on the skin
    c. Clean the area with water and mild soap as directed by the nurse
    d. Wipe with tissues until clean

56. You should wear gloves when testing a stool for occult blood to
    a. prevent contact with body fluids and substances.
    b. prevent contaminating the specimen.
    c. maintain a sterile specimen.
    d. prevent contact with chemicals used in the test.

Labelling

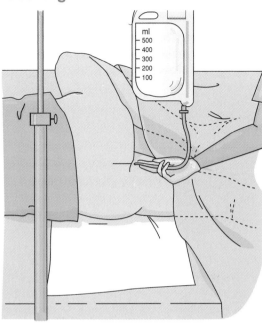

57. a. How high above the anus should the bag hang?

    _____

    b. How high above the mattress should bag hang?

    _____

58. How far should the tube be inserted into the rectum?

    _____

59. Identify the position of the person.

    _____

Independent Learning Activities

1. Do you ever have difficulty regulating your own bowel elimination? Answer these questions about how you treat problems with bowel elimination.
   - What causes you to have problems with bowel elimination? Foods? Illness? Stress? Inactivity?
   - What methods have you used to treat problems with bowel elimination? Diet? Medication?
   - How do youeel when problems with bowel elimination occur? What type of physical discomfort occurs? Emotional distress?
   - How do problems with bowel elimination affect your appetite? Sleep and rest? Energy level? Mood?
   - What effect does a problem with bowel elimination have on your life? How does it affect your participation in work and leisure activities?
   - How can you relate your personal experience to the feelings and concerns of a person you are caring for who has problems with bowel elimination?

2. Do you know someone who has a colostomy or ileostomy? If you feel comfortable with the person, ask these questions to better understand the problems the person has daily.
   - How long has the person had the ostomy? Is it permanent or temporary?
   - What problems has the person experienced in learning to live with the ostomy? How have friends, family, and others reacted to knowing the person has an ostomy?
   - What has been the hardest adjustment? What has been the easiest?
   - What type of pouch is being used? What other types were tried? What are the advantages of the type being used?
   - How much time is required each day to care for the ostomy? What is the person's schedule to care for the ostomy?
   - How expensive is the equipment used?
   - What leisure activities does the person have? Did the person have to change or give up any activities due to the colostomy? What changes occurred in the person's body image?

Common Diseases and Conditions

Fill-In-the-Blanks

1. List any six early warning signs of cancer?

   a. _____

   b. _____

   c. _____

   d. _____

   e. _____

   f. _____

   g. _____

2. Why are special skin care procedures often ordered for a person receiving radiation therapy for cancer?

   _____

3. What side effects of radiation therapy cause a person with cancer to have special needs in his/her care?

   a. _____

   b. _____

   c. _____

   d. _____

   e. _____

   f. _____

4. Elevated toilet sets are helpful to a person with osteoarthritis when the person has limited

   _____.

5. Why does a person with osteoarthritis have more pain when standing and walking?

   _____.

6. What treatments are used to relieve pain and stiffness for a person with osteoarthritis?

   a. _____

   b. _____

   c. _____

   d. _____

   e. _____

7. What type of arthritis occurs in children?

   _____

8. What are the goals in treating rheumatoid arthritis?

   a. _____

   b. _____

   c. _____

9. When a person has osteoporosis, a fracture can

   occur when _____

   _____

   because the bones are very brittle.

10. A child falls and has signs and symptoms of a fracture. These would include:

    a. _____

    b. _____

    c. _____

    d. _____

    e. _____

11. These are signs and symptoms that should be reported immediately if they occur to a person with a cast. What could be happening to cause each of the symptoms?

    a. Pain

    _____

    b. Swelling/tight cast

    _____

    c. Pale skin

    _____

    d. Cyanosis

    _____

    e. Odour

    _____

    f. Inability to move toes or fingers

    _____

g. Numbness

   _____

h. Temperature changes

   _____

i. Drainage on or under cast

   _____

j. Chills, fever, nausea, vomiting

   _____

12. Aside from reporting the symptoms above, what other rules should you follow when caring for a person with a cast?

    a. _____

    b. _____

    c. _____

    d. _____

13. Why are older people at higher risk for serious problems after a hip fracture?

    a. _____

    b. _____

14. When you care for a person with a hip fracture, what measures are important for you to follow?

    a. _____

    b. _____

    c. _____

    d. _____

    e. _____

    f. _____

15. When gangrene causes an extremity to be amputated, what areas of the person's life may be affected?

    a. _____

    b. _____

    c. _____

16. If you are caring for a person who has had a stroke, you might observe effects such as

    a. _____

    b. _____

    c. _____

    d. _____

    e. _____

    f. _____

    g. _____

17. What measures would be helpful to use when you care for a person with a stroke?

    a. _____

    b. _____

    c. _____

    d. _____

    e. _____

    f. _____

    g. _____

18. Why are exercise and physical therapy ordered for a person with Parkinson's disease?

    _____

19. A person with Parkinson's disease may need assistance with:

    a. _____

    b. _____

    c. _____

    d. _____

20. Infants and children may suffer brain damage from head injuries caused by

    a. _____

    b. _____

    c. _____

    d. _____

21. A person with chronic obstructive pulmonary disease (COPD) must stop

    _____.

22. A person with emphysema can breathe more easily if he/she is allowed to sit

    _____.

23. Why is it important to control asthma and prevent asthma attacks?

    _____.

24. How can you help the person with pneumonia to breathe more easily and be more comfortable?

    a. _____

    b. _____

    c. _____

25. How is the tuberculosis bacteria spread?

    _____

26. What precautions to prevent infection should be used when caring for a person with tuberculosis?

    a. _____

    b. _____

27. When caring for a person with tuberculosis, how should you dispose of tissues?

    a. In the home

    _____

    b. In a health care facility

    _____

28. How do these risk factors affect hypertension?

    a. Age

    _____

    b. Atherosclerosis

    _____

    c. Ethnicity

    _____

    d. Family history

    _____

    e. Obesity

    _____

    f. Stress

    _____

    g. Cigarette smoking

    _____

    h. Alcohol

    _____

29. What damage can hypertension do to other body organs?

    a. _____

    b. _____

    c. _____

    d. _____

30. Which risk factors of coronary artery disease can be changed by the person through lifestyle changes?

    a. _____

    b. _____

    c. _____

    d. _____

    e. _____

31. What signs and symptoms would tell you a person is experiencing angina pectoris?

    a. _____

    b. _____

    c. _____

    d. _____

32. How is pain from angina relieved or avoided?

    a. _____

    b. _____

    c. _____

    d. _____

    e. _____

    f. _____

33. If a person is having a myocardial infarction, his/her signs and symptoms may include

    a. _____

    b. _____

    c. _____

    d. _____

    e. _____

    f. _____

    g. _____

34. If a person has heart failure, what signs and symptoms occur when these organs do not get enough blood?

    a. Brain

    _____

    b. Kidneys

    _____

    c. Skin

    _____

35. What measures could you use when caring for a person with heart failure?

    a. _____

    b. _____

    c. _____

    d. _____

    e. _____

36. Why are older people with heart failure at risk for skin breakdown?

    _____

37. What can you do to help prevent any skin breakdown?

    _____

38. If you are caring for a person who has renal calculi, you should encourage the person to drink about

    _____ per day.

39. When you are caring for a person with acute renal failure, the care plan is likely to include

    a. _____

    b. _____

    c. _____

    d. _____

    e. _____

    f. _____

    g. _____

40. With acute renal failure, recovery may take

    _____.

41. With chronic renal failure, the nephrons of the kidneys are

    _____.

42. Dialysis is done with chronic renal failure to remove

    _____.

43. What measures are used to care for a person in chronic renal failure?

    a. _____

    b. _____

    c. _____

d. _____

e. _____

f. _____

g. _____

h. _____

44. List the three types of diabetes mellitus and the age or situation when each type usually occurs.

a. _____

b. _____

c. _____

45. Complications of diabetes mellitus are

_____

46. Why is good foot care very important for a diabetic?

_____

47. What are the signs and symptoms of hepatitis?

a. _____

b. _____

c. _____

d. _____

e. _____

f. _____

g. _____

h. _____

48. To protect yourself from contracting hepatitis, you

use _____.

The most important way to prevent the spread of hepatitis is practising

_____.

49. AIDS is spread by:

a. _____

b. _____

c. _____

d. _____

e. _____

50. Signs and symptoms of AIDS related to the following include

a. Skin _____

_____

b. Mouth and neck _____

_____

c. Mental status _____

_____

d. Digestive system _____

_____

51. Why does a person with AIDS often develop other diseases?

_____

52. STDs may enter the body through many body areas such as the

_____

53. The use of condoms will help prevent the spread of

_____

54. What signs and symptoms may occur with both hypoglycemia and hyperglycemia?

 a. _____

 b. _____

 c. _____

 d. _____

 e. _____

 f. _____

 g. _____

 h. _____

55 What disease do the following signs and symptoms describe?
 - Unusual mass or swelling
 - Unexplained paleness or loss of energy
 - Sudden tendency to bruise
 - Persistent localized pain
 - Frequent headaches especially with vomiting

_____

56. What disease do the following signs and symptoms describe?
 - The alveoli become enlarged
 - Walls of the alveoli become less elastic
 - Some air remains trapped in the alveoli during expiration
 - Shortness of breath and "smoker's cough"
 - Barrel chest

_____

57. What disease do the following signs and symptoms describe?
 - Blurred or double vision
 - Numbness and tingling
 - Muscle weakness
 - Difficult speech
 - Dizziness, poor coordination
 - Bladder problems

_____

58. What disease do the following signs and symptoms describe?
 - Sudden weakness or numbness on one side of body
 - Dimness or loss of vision
 - Loss of speech or trouble talking
 - Loss of face control
 - Unexplained dizziness
 - Impaired vision

_____

59. What disease do the following signs and symptoms describe?
 - Mask-like facial expression
 - Tremors, pill-rolling movements of the fingers
 - Shuffling gait, impaired balance
 - Stooped posture, stiff muscles
 - Slurred or monotone speech
 - Drooling

_____

Matching

Match the COPD disorder with the symptom or physical effect related to that disorder.

60. _____ Person develops barrel chest

61. _____ Mucus and inflamed breathing passages obstruct airflow

62. _____ Walls of alveoli are less elastic

a. Chronic bronchitis

b. Emphysema

Match the symptom with either hypoglycemia or hyperglycemia.

63. _____ Trembling

64. _____ Nausea and vomiting

65. _____ Cold, clammy skin

66. _____ Flushed face

67. _____ Tiredness and fatigue

68. _____ Dizziness

69. _____ Dry skin

70. _____ Sweating

71. _____ Slow, laboured breathing

a. Hypoglycemia

b. Hyperglycemia

True or False

Circle T for true or F for false. Rewrite all false statements to make them true.

72. T F Joint stiffness occurs in osteoarthritis with activity and range-of-motion exercises.

_____

_____

73. T F Rheumatoid arthritis affects only the large weight-bearing joints.

_____

_____

74. T F Rheumatoid arthritis in children can affect growth and development.

_____

_____

75. T F Arthroplasty is done to cure arthritis.

_____

_____

76. **T** **F** You can help to prevent osteoporosis by taking calcium and having a regular exercise program.

_____

_____

77. **T** **F** When turning and repositioning a person with osteoporosis, you should move him/her quickly to prevent fractures.

_____

_____

78. **T** **F** You must protect a person with osteoporosis from falls because he/she is at high risk for joint injuries.

_____

_____

79. **T** **F** An infant who has a fracture may be a victim of child abuse.

_____

_____

80. **T** **F** Phantom limb pains occur when a person has an amputation.

_____

_____

81. **T** **F** A stroke occurs when brain cells get too much oxygen and too many nutrients.

_____

_____

82. **T** **F** All people with Parkinson's disease will have impaired mental function but should be treated with dignity and respect.

_____

_____

83. **T** **F** Multiple sclerosis is a short-term, acute disease.

_____

_____

84. **T** **F** A person with COPD is at risk for respiratory infections.

_____

_____

85. **T** **F** Tuberculosis is spread by contact with infectious materials.

_____

_____

86. **T** **F** You can contract tuberculosis through casual contact with a person who has the disease.

_____

_____

87. **T** **F** Angina pectoris occurs when vessels narrow and the heart pumps with more force.

_____

_____

88. **T** **F** Activity will usually relieve angina pain in 3 to 15 minutes.

_____

_____

89. **T** **F** A common term for a myocardial infarction is _heart attack_.

_____

_____

90. **T** **F** The goal of cardiac rehabilitation after a myocardial infarction is to prevent another attack.

_____

_____

91. **T** **F** When a person has renal calculi, you should strain the urine.

_____

_____

92. **T** **F** When a person has chronic renal failure, only the renal system is affected.

_____

_____

93. **T** **F** If a person is vomiting, you need to use only Standard Precautions.

_____

_____

94. **T** **F** A person who has HIV, but has not developed AIDS, cannot infect others with the virus.

_____

_____

Circle the Correct Answer

95. If a person with rheumatoid arthritis tells you she has wrist pain, you would be correct to expect the pain to be
    a. in the dominant hand.
    b. in the nondominant hand.
    c. in both wrists.
    d. None of the above.

96. Which of the following is *not* a cause of osteoporosis?
    a. Lack of estrogen
    b. Regular exercise
    c. Lack of dietary calcium
    d. Bed rest and immobility

97. When caring for a person who had a hip replacement 5 weeks ago, which of these activities would not be allowed?
    a. Abduction of the affected leg
    b. Using an abductor splint or pillow between the legs when in bed
    c. Crossing the legs when sitting
    d. Using a shower chair for bathing

98. Gangrene can occur because of
    a. joint immobility and inflammation.
    b. infection, injuries, and decreased circulation.
    c. poor body alignment and positioning.
    d. porous, brittle bones.

99. A transient ischemic attack (TIA)
    a. is another name for a stroke.
    b. occurs when blood supply to the brain is disrupted for a short period.
    c. occurs when blood pressure is elevated.
    d. occurs when there is high sugar in the blood.

100. The goal of rehabilitation with a spinal cord injury is
    a. to return to all normal activities.
    b. to learn to function at the person's highest level.
    c. to regain use of arms and legs.
    d. to prevent further injury.

101. You are caring for a person who has angina and you find a bottle of tablets marked "Nitroglycerin" at the bedside. You should
    a. place them in a locked cabinet.
    b. tell the nurse.
    c. give them to the family to take home.
    d. make sure they remain where the person put them.

102. Which of these measures would *not* be included in the treatment of a person with chronic heart failure?
    a. A diet high in salt
    b. Oxygen
    c. Drugs to strengthen the heart
    d. A semi-Fowler's or Fowler's position for easier breathing

103. Childhood communicable diseases are most commonly transmitted by
    a. airborne or direct contact with respiratory secretions.
    b. direct contact with feces.
    c. direct contact with skin lesions.
    d. contact with a carrier.

Labelling

104. Colour the area that would be paralyzed if the person had a cervical spine injury.

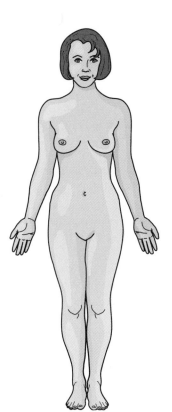

105. Colour the area that would be paralyzed if the person had a lumbar spine injury.

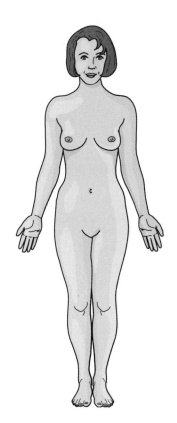

Independent Learning Activities

1. Many people have had a fracture at some time during their life. If you have had a broken bone, answer the questions based on your experience.
   - How did it feel? Did you know it was broken right away or several hours or days later? How much pain did you have?
   - What treatment was done? A cast? Surgery? Pins, plates, screws, traction?
   - What effect did the fracture have on your day-to-day activities? Work? Schooling? Leisure activities?
   - What accommodations were needed to carry out ADLs? Toileting? Bathing? Dressing?
   - How was mobility affected? Ambulation? Sitting in a car? Driving a car?
   - What discomfort or pain did you experience during the healing process? With the cast? With any surgical incision?
   - What long-range problems occurred because of this injury? Periodic pain? Limited mobility?

2. If you have never had a fracture, try this experiment to get a small sample of how the fracture may interfere with your life. Make an immobilizer for your leg. Use one of the methods suggested or devise your own immobilizer.
   - Use four pieces of sturdy cardboard that are long enough to reach from the ankle to mid-thigh. Place on the front, back, and sides of the leg.
   - Use several thicknesses of newspaper or magazines and wrap around the leg to immobilize the knee and ankle.
   - Secure the immobilizer with an elastic bandage or soft cloth strips.
   - After the immobilizer is in place, leave it on for 1 to 2 hours and go about your normal routine. Answer the questions about what you experienced.
   - How much did the "cast" interfere with your routine?
   - What problems occurred because of the cast?
   - How did you feel when you were in the cast? Awkward? As if everyone were looking at you?

3. Try these experiments to understand how these diseases affect the body or the person.
   Osteoporosis: Fold a piece of standard 22 X 28 cm (8 1/2 X 11 inch) paper in half, in half again and in half a third time. (It will now be about 3.5 X 28 cm). Now try to break it in half; pull it from either end to break it. What happens? Unfold the paper once and cut several holes along the edges. If necessary, unfold it again to carry out this step. This will make the paper porous, much like bone becomes with osteoporosis. Refold the paper to the original 3.5 X 28 cm size and attempt to break it in half or pull it apart from the ends. What happens this time?
   Coronary artery disease: Use a straw to drink water. Now, put small pieces of paper towel into the end of the straw and try to drink through it. What happens? Keep adding more paper towel to the straw and try to draw fluid through the straw. How does this relate to coronary artery disease?

4. Consider the following situation. Answer the questions about how you would respond to this information.

   SITUATION: Your doctor has just told you that you have cancer and will probably live only 6 months.
   - How do you think you would react immediately? After a few days?
   - What changes would you make in your life? Why?
   - What would be your biggest concern? Why?
   - What would you want to do with the time you had? With whom would you want to spend the time?
   - With whom would you share the information about your diagnosis?
   - How would you respond to others who offered sympathy or assistance? Why would you respond in this way?
   - How would you like others to treat you at this time? Why?

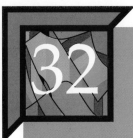

Rehabilitation and Restorative Care

Matching

Match the following words with the correct definitions.

1. _____ Process of restoring a person to the highest possible level of function

2. _____ Self-care activities performed to remain independent

4. _____ Helps a person regain health and strength

a. Activities of daily living

b. Independence

c. Rehabilitation

Fill-In-the-Blanks

4. The following goals of rehabilitation are common:

   a. _____

   b. _____

   c. _____

   d. _____

5. The goal of a prosthesis is _____
   _____.

6. Examples of orthoses are

   a. _____

   b. _____

   c. _____

   d. _____

7. Rehabilitation can occur in different settings. List some of the settings.

   a. _____

   b. _____

   c. _____

   d. _____

8. Common health problems requiring rehabilitation are

   a. _____

   b. _____

   c. _____

   d. _____

e. _____

f. _____

g. _____

h. _____

9. Why is good skin care important in rehabilitation?

_____

10. How can an electric toothbrush help a person with a disability become more independent?

_____

_____

11. How can you improve the quality of life for a person with a disability?

a. Right to privacy

_____

b. Preferences

_____

c. Dignity

_____

d. Safety

_____

e. Independence

_____

12. Why is the home assessed by the rehabilitation team before a person goes home?

_____

True or False

Circle **T** *for true or* **F** *for false. Rewrite all false statements to make them true.*

13. **T   F**   A disability does not affect the person's psychological well-being. It is only a physical problem.

_____

_____

14. **T   F**   Rehabilitation begins by preventing complications.

_____

_____

15. **T   F**   Rehabilitation often takes less time in older persons than in other age groups.

_____

_____

16. **T   F**   Health care workers as well as the person and family members are part of the rehabilitation team.

_____

_____

17. **T   F**   When the health care team sets goals for the person, they can never be changed.

_____

_____

Independent Learning Activities

1. Role-play the situation with a classmate. Answer the questions about how you felt when you played Mrs. Leeds to understand how a person with a disability feels. Use your nondominant hand to attempt the activities she must do.

    SITUATION: Mrs. Leeds is 62 and had a cerebrovascular accident last month. She has weakness on her dominant side and has been admitted to a rehabilitation unit to relearn activities of daily living (ADLs). She is practising eating by using a spoon to place fluids and food in her mouth. She is also learning to button clothing.
    *   How well could you hold the spoon with your nondominant hand? What problems did you having controlling the spoon?
    *   How rapidly could you eat? What type of food was easier to eat?
    *   How well were you able to button your clothing? What techniques did you find that made you more successful?
    *   How did this experience make you feel? How will it affect the way you interact with people who have similar disabilities?

2. With your instructor's permission, borrow a wheelchair from your school to use for 1 to 2 hours. Have a classmate push you around in the chair in a grocery store or mall. You must stay in the chair for the entire time to experience the feelings of a person who must use a wheelchair. Use a wheelchair-accessible bathroom during this experience.
    *   How comfortable was the wheelchair? Did you use any special padding or cushion in the seat?
    *   What difficulties were encountered moving about? Doorways? Steps? Aisles? Crowds? How did you deal with any difficulties?
    *   How accessible was the specially equipped bathroom? How much room was available for you to transfer from the wheelchair to the toilet?
    *   How did other people treat you? How many spoke to you? How many directed conversations to your classmate and avoided you?
    *   How did this experience make you feel? How will it affect the way you interact with a person in a wheelchair?

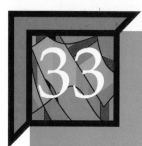

33

Mental Health Disorders

Fill-In-the-Blanks

1. What are some of the causes of mental health disorders?

   a. _____

   _____

   b. _____

   _____

   c. _____

   _____

   d. _____

   _____

2. The various forms of psychotherapy include

   a. _____

   b. _____

   c. _____

   d. _____

3. A person suffering from schizophrenia may exhibit the following behaviours:

   a. _____

   b. _____

   c. _____

   d. _____

4. Signs and symptoms of depression include

   a. _____

   b. _____

   c. _____

   d. _____

5. An obsession is a

   _____.

6. A compulsion is

   _____.

7. Why does a person act on an obsessive idea?

   _____.

8. If a person believes he/she is the prime minister of Canada, what type of false belief is present?

   _____.

9. What are the two extremes of a bipolar disorder?

   _____.

10. An older person has the following symptoms: fatigue, slow or unreliable memory, agitation, and thoughts of death. It may be that he/she is suffering from

    _____.

11. A person with _____ craves food. After eating, the person induces

    _____.

12. Why does a person with bulimia take diuretics?

    _____.

    _____.

13. What are the following statements describing?
    - Thinking and behaviour are disturbed
    - Delusions and hallucinations are present
    - Difficulty relating to others and the world

    _____

14. What are the following statements describing?
    - Vague, uneasy feelings
    - Feels sense of danger or harm
    - Occurs in response to stress
    - Unaware of source of uneasy feeling

    _____

15. What are the following statements describing?
    - Has extreme mood swings
    - At times feels very sad, lonely, worthless
    - Tends to run in families
    - At times has much energy and is excited

    _____

16. What are the following statements describing?
    - Abusive
    - Paranoid
    - Distrusts others
    - Irresponsible

    _____

Circle the Correct Answer

17. Which of these may cause mental health disorders?
    a. Inability to cope with stress
    b. Chemical imbalances in body
    c. Characteristics inherited from parents
    d. All of the above

18. Which of the following is an example of an unhealthy coping mechanism?
    a. Going for a walk
    b. Exercising
    c. Chain smoking
    d. Having a piece of cake with a meal

19. An older person may not be diagnosed for depression because
    a. it rarely occurs in an older person.
    b. treatment of physical problems is more important in the older person.
    c. the older person may be thought to have dementia.
    d. it is usually mild and does not require treatment.

20. Which of these would be present if the person has delusions of persecution?
    a. Seeing, hearing, or feeling something that is not there
    b. Not sleeping or taking time to tend to self-care needs
    c. Believing that one is mistreated, abused, or harassed
    d. Having poor judgment and morals and lacking ethics

21. When a girl has anorexia nervosa, which of these behaviours is she likely to display?
    a. Diets even though she becomes emaciated
    b. Withdraws from the world and shows no interest in others
    c. Retreats to behaviours of a younger-aged child
    d. Has delusions or hallucinations

22. Which of these substances can be abused?
    a. Legal drugs
    b. Illegal drugs
    c. Alcohol
    d. All of the above

Independent Learning Activities

1. Try this experiment with a group of classmates. Make up labels with various roles for "staff members" and "mentally ill" people. A list is provided, but you may add or subtract according to the size of your group. Make sure that the group includes a mixture of people with mental health problems and staff or visitors.

Doctor	A person with bipolar disorder
Nurse	A person with delusions of grandeur
Visitor	A person with obsessive-compulsive disorder
Support worker	A person with schizophrenia with paranoia
Recreational therapist	A person with hallucinations
Dietician	A person with anorexia nervosa

Attach a label to each person so that he or she cannot read it. (It may be placed on the back or the forehead.) Have everyone move about the group and talk to each other based on how the person thinks he or she should approach the person with a certain "label." Continue the experiment for about 15 minutes and then use the questions to guide a group discussion.

- How did you feel talking to a person with a mental health disorder?
- How were the people with a mental health disorder approached? How quickly were the "mentally ill" able to sense that this was their label? What cues did they receive from others?
- How quickly did "staff members" recognize the label they had? What cues did they receive from others?
- In what ways did the approach of others cause people to respond in a way expected? Did the people with mental health problems show signs of the illness based on the reaction of others?
- What did the group learn about approaching a person with a mental health problem?

2. Consider this situation and answer the questions concerning how you would feel about caring for a person with a mental health problem.

SITUATION: Mrs. Cross, 65, is a patient in an acute care hospital with a diagnosis of pneumonia. The nurse tells you Mrs. Cross has a history of schizophrenia. You are assigned to provide AM care for Mrs. Cross.

- How would you approach Mrs. Cross when you entered her room? How would your knowledge about her mental health problem affect your initial contact with her?
- What would you do if Mrs. Cross told you she saw an elephant in the room? What would you say to her?
- How would you react if Mrs. Cross told you that she owned Disney World and went there free any time she wanted? How would you respond?
- How would you provide good oral hygiene if Mrs. Cross refused to cooperate because she was sure the staff was trying to poison her? What could you try that might be helpful?
- What would you do if Mrs. Cross curled up in a tight ball and refused to talk or cooperate during AM care? What could you do to maintain her hygiene?
- How would you feel about caring for a person with abnormal behaviour? Why?

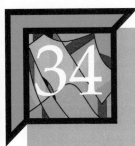

Confusion and Dementia

Circle the Correct Answer

1. Which of the following interventions would *not* help when caring for a confused person?
   a. State your name and show your name tag
   b. Give very detailed answers to questions to help the person understand
   c. Call the person by name each time you are in contact with him or her
   d. Encourage the person to wear glasses and a hearing aid if needed

2. Which of these is helpful when a person with Alzheimer's disease is agitated?
   a. Keep the person in a calm, quiet environment
   b. Complete care very quickly
   c. Place in a darkened room
   d. Take to an area with music, activity, and people

3. How can a person who wanders be protected?
   a. Make sure the person receives medication to calm him/her down
   b. Restrain the person to prevent movement or wandering
   c. Go with the person who insists on going outside
   d. Explain to the person why going outside is not possible

4. What service is *not* offered by the Alzheimer's disease support group?
   a. Advice and ideas about caring for the person with Alzheimer's disease
   b. Assistance with financial needs
   c. A place to share anger and frustration
   d. Support and encouragement to family

Matching

Match each statement with one of the two disorders given.

5. _____ May get lost in familiar places

6. _____ Can occur after surgery

7. _____ Anger, restlessness, depression, and irritability may occur

8. _____ May be caused by losses of hearing and sight

9. _____ Progressive loss of cognitive and social funtions

a. Confusion

b. Dementia

161

Match the symptom of dementia to the stage where it usually first occurs.

10. _____ Restlessness that increases during evening hours

11. _____ Cannot walk or sit

12. _____ Less outgoing and less interested in things

13. _____ Forgets recent events

14. _____ Does not recognize family members

15. _____ May say same thing over and over

16. _____ Cannot tell difference between hot and cold

17. _____ Totally incontinent of urine and feces

18. _____ Disoriented to time and place

19. _____ Cannot communicate

20. _____ Has difficulty following directions

a. Stage 1

b. Stage 2

c. Stage 3

Match the area of concern for people with dementia with a strategy to give care in that area.

21. _____ Follow facility policy for locking doors and windows

22. _____ Provide plastic eating and drinking utensils

23. _____ Tell him/her that you will provide protection from harm

24. _____ Give consistent responses

25. _____ Provide for person's food and fluid needs

26. _____ Try bathing the person when he/she is calm

27. _____ Play music and show movies from the person's past

28. _____ Make sure person wears an ID bracelet at all times

29. _____ Dim lights and play soft music to help calm the person

30. _____ Approach person in a calm, quiet manner

31. _____ Store personal care items in a safe place

32. _____ Use touch to calm and reassure person

a. Environment

b. Communication

c. Safety

d. Wandering

e. Sundowning

f. Hallucinations and delusions

g. Basic needs

33. _____ Keep personal care items where person can see them

34. _____ Do not argue with person who wants to leave

35. _____ Have equipment ready for any procedure ahead of time

36. _____ Remove dangerous appliances and power tools from home

37. _____ Make sure person has eaten because hunger can increase restlessness

Fill-In-the-Blanks

38. What are the early warning signs of dementia?

  a. _____

  b. _____

  c. _____

  d. _____

  e. _____

  f. _____

  g. _____

39. Delirium is common in _____

  with _____ illnesses.

40. The risk of Alzheimer's disease increases after the age of

  _____.

41. Why is a person with dementia in danger of having accidents?

  _____

42. List some of the behaviours associated with early stage dementia.

  a. _____

  b. _____

  c. _____

  d. _____

  e. _____

  f. _____

  g. _____

43. These are problems that occur with dementia. Describe each one or the behaviour that is displayed with the problem.

  a. Wandering _____

  _____

  b. Sundowning _____

  _____

  c. Hallucinations _____

  _____

  d. Delusions _____

  _____

  e. Catastrophic reaction _____

  _____

  f. Agitation and restlessness _____

  _____

  g. Aggression and combativeness _____

  _____

h. Screaming _____

_____

i. Abnormal sexual behaviour _____

_____

j. Repetitive behaviours _____

_____

44. How can a caregiver cause agitation and restlessness?

_____

45. List ways caregivers help calm a person with dementia who screams?

a. _____

b. _____

c. _____

d. _____

46. How can you help the person with Alzheimer's disease who displays abnormal sexual behaviour?

_____

_____

47. What are reasons why sundowning may occur in a person with Alzheimer's disease?

a. _____

b. _____

c. _____

48. What response may occur if the person with Alzheimer's disease has too much stimuli at one time?

_____

49. What are reasons why a family usually decides to place a person with Alzheimer's disease in a long-term care facility?

a. _____

b. _____

c. _____

d. _____

50. Complete these statements that relate to caring for a confused person.

a. Face the person and _____

_____.

b. Explain what _____

_____.

c. Give short, simple _____

_____.

d. Keep calendars and clocks with _____

_____.

e. Allow the person to place _____

_____

f. Ask _____

questions. Allow enough time _____

_____.

g. Maintain _____

_____ atmosphere.

h. Remind the person of _____

_____.

51. How can you maintain the day-night cycle for a confused person?

    a. _____

    b. _____

    c. _____

52. What can you do to maintain a confused person's routine?

    _____

    Why is this important?

    _____

    _____

53. What is meant by the "sandwich generation?"

    _____

54. Why are locks placed at the top or bottom of a door to prevent wandering?

    _____

55. Why is it ineffective to argue or try to reason with a person with Alzheimer's disease?

    _____

True or False

Circle T for true or F for false. Rewrite all false statements to make them true.

56. **T   F**   Only tell a confused person the date and time once a day.

    _____

    _____

57. **T   F**   When caring for confused people, you should provide newspapers and magazines and provide access to TV and radio.

    _____

    _____

58. **T   F**   Rearrange furniture or the belongings of a confused person.

    _____

    _____

59. **T   F**   Delirium is a permanent, chronic mental confusion.

    _____

    _____

60. **T   F**   Delirium is an emergency.

    _____

    _____

61. **T   F**   Repetitious behaviour is usually harmless, and the person can be allowed to continue with the actions.

    _____

    _____

62. **T   F**   People with Alzheimer's disease can control their behaviours of forgetfulness, incontinence, agitation, or rudeness with direction.

    _____

    _____

63. **T   F**   Alzheimer's disease progresses slowly at a predictable rate in all people.

    _____

    _____

Independent Learning Activities

1. Consider the situation and answer the questions about how you would feel.

   SITUATION: Imagine you are in a strange country where people talk to you, but you do not understand what they are saying. They use strange tools to eat and you cannot figure out how to use them. They try to feed you food you do not recognize. Sometimes these people seem friendly and caring, but at other times they become angry because you are not doing what they ask you to do. You become frightened when they try to remove your clothes and take you in a room to shower you. You become frightened and upset because you do not know what will happen next. At times other strangers come to your room and bring gifts. They talk kindly to you, but you do not know them. They seem upset when you do not respond to their gifts and gestures. The doors and windows in this country are all locked, and you cannot find a way out so that you can go home.
   - How does this situation relate to the information in this chapter?
   - How would you react if you were the person in this situation? Why?
   - What methods might you use to try to communicate with the person in this situation?
   - Why would the person want to go home? What does "home" mean to him or her?
   - How will this exercise help you when you care for a person who is confused?

2. Consider the situation and answer the questions about how you would care for a person who has dementia.

   SITUATION: You are assigned to care for Mr. Myers, 85, who has Alzheimer's disease. He often wanders from room to room and tries to open the outside doors. He frequently becomes agitated and restless, especially in the evening. Most of the time, Mr. Myers is unable to feed himself and is often incontinent. He keeps repeating, "Help me, help me" all day long.
   - How do you feel about caring for a person like this? Frightened? Angry? Impatient?
   - How do you deal with your feelings so that you can give care to the person?
   - At what stage of Alzheimer's disease is Mr. Myers? What signs and symptoms support your answer?
   - Why would it be ineffective to remind Mr. Myers of the date and time during your shift?
   - Why is this a good technique with some confused people and not with others?
   - Why does Mr. Myers become more agitated toward evening? What is this called?
   - What methods could you use to make sure Mr. Myers receives the care needed to maintain good personal hygiene? How could you get him to cooperate or participate in his care?
   - What parts of Mr. Myers' behaviour would be most difficult for you to tolerate?
   - What would you do if you found yourself becoming irritated and angry with Mr. Myers?
   - What information in this chapter has helped you to understand people like Mr. Myers better? How will this information help you to give better care to these people and to maintain their quality of life?

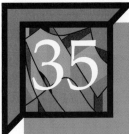

Speech and Language Disorders

Fill-In-the-Blanks

1. What can cause speech and language disorders?

   a. _____

   b. _____

   c. _____

   d. _____

   e. _____

2. List the three basic types of aphasia, and briefly describe the differences.

   a. _____

   _____

   _____

   b. _____

   _____

   _____

   c. _____

   _____

   _____

3. Apraxia of speech means _____.

   People with this disorder _____

   _____.

4. Dysarthria means _____.

   People with this disorder _____

   _____.

5. What are some of the emotions people with speech and language disorders may experience?

   a. _____

   b. _____

   c. _____

   d. _____

6. How do you provide compassionate care to clients who have speech or language disorders?

   a. _____

   _____

   _____

   b. _____

   _____

   _____

   c. _____

   _____

   _____

d. _____

_____

_____

7. Some guidelines to effective communication with clients with speech or language disorders are

a. _____

b. _____

c. _____

d. _____

e. _____

f. _____

*Circle **T** for true or **F** for false. Rewrite all the false statements to make them true.*

8. **T   F**   Most people with dementia have apraxia.

_____

_____

9. **T   F**   Some people with aphasia cannot understand the message.

_____

_____

10. **T   F**   People with expressive aphasia are not aware of their mistakes when speaking.

_____

_____

11. **T   F**   Dysarthria is caused by weakness in the muscles used for speech.

_____

_____

12. **T   F**   Relations between family members are not affected when someone has a speech disorder.

_____

_____

13. **T   F**   Shopping and cooking are not affected when someone has a communication problem.

_____

_____

14. **T   F**   Because you don't need to spend time on communication, you can take less time giving care to someone who can't speak.

_____

_____

15. **T   F**   It is a help to the client to finish words for him/her.

_____

_____

16. **T   F**   Use positive statements rather than negative statements.

_____

_____

17. **T   F**   Aphasia is seldom permanent.

_____

_____

Circle the Correct Answer

18. When you are caring for a person who thinks clearly but cannot speak, which type of aphasia is the person likely to have?

a. Expressive aphasia
b. Receptive aphasia
c. Expressive-receptive aphasia
d. Hemiplegia

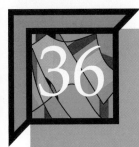

Hearing and Vision Problems

Matching

Match the terms related to hearing and vision problems with the correct definition.

1. _____ Dizziness

2. _____ Ringing in the ears

3. _____ Method of writing using raised dots

4. _____ Infection of the middle ear

a. Otitis media

b. Tinnitus

c. Vertigo

d. Braille

Communication Practice

5. Use the sign language chart in the textbook to identify what the person is telling you.

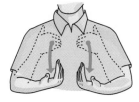 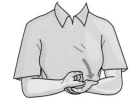

_____

Fill-In-the-Blanks

6. Explain why the following behaviours may occur in people with hearing problems?

a. Avoids social situations

_____

b. Controls conversations

_____

c. Fatigue, frustration, irritability

_____

7. What guidelines will help you to communicate better with a person with hearing loss?

   a. _____

   b. _____

   c. _____

   d. _____

   e. _____

   f. _____

   g. _____

   h. _____

   i. _____

8. What should you do if a hearing aid does not seem to work properly?

   a. _____

   b. _____

   c. _____

   d. _____

9. What should you do to clean and store eyeglasses?

   a. Cleaning

   _____

   b. Storage

   _____

10. How do you clean an artificial eye?

    a. _____

    b. _____

    c. _____

    d. _____

e. _____

f. _____

g. _____

h. _____

11. If you see a person with a white cane with a red tip or a guide dog, you should recognize that person is

    _____.

12. List measures to practise when caring for a person with vision loss.

    a. _____

    b. _____

    c. _____

    d. _____

    e. _____

    f. _____

13. What disease do the following statements describe?
    - In this disease, pressure within the eye is increased.
    - It has a gradual or sudden onset.
    - The signs and symptoms include tunnel vision, blurred vision, and blue-green halos around lights.
    - With a sudden onset, there also is severe eye pain, nausea, and vomiting.

    _____

14. What disease do the following statements describe?
    - This disease involves increased fluid in the inner ear.
    - Symptoms are vertigo, tinnitus, and hearing loss.

    _____

15. What disorder do the following statements describe?
    - In this disorder, the lens becomes opaque.
    - A gradual blurring and dimming of vision occurs.
    - It can occur in one or both eyes.
    - Aging is the most common cause.

    _____

Circle the Correct Answers

16. Which disorder may cause vertigo?
    a. Glaucoma
    b. Otitis media
    c. Ménière's disease
    d. Cataracts

17. Which of these signs may indicate a person has a hearing loss?
    a. Speaking very softly
    b. Asking for words to be repeated
    c. Pronouncing words very clearly
    d. Answering questions appropriately while watching TV

18. What is the most common cause of blindness in people over 50?
    a. Cataracts
    b. Age-related macular degeneration
    c. Vertigo
    d. Otitis media

19. Which of these is *not* a responsibility of a support worker?
    a. Check the battery position in a hearing aid
    b. Clean eyeglasses with warm water
    c. Assist person to remove an artificial eye
    d. Remove wax from the ear canal

20. When a person is legally blind it means he/she
    a. cannot sense light and has no usable vision.
    b. can sense some light, but has no usable vision.
    c. has some usable vision but cannot read newsprint.
    d. sees at 6 m what a person with normal vision sees at 60 m.

Independent Learning Activities

1. Cover your ears so that you cannot hear clearly. Use one of these methods or one that you devise.
   - Commercial earplugs
   - Cotton plugs in ears
   - Cover ears with earmuffs or similar devices

   Keep your ears covered and hearing muffled for at least 1 hour as you go about your daily activities. A wise student will *not* wear earplugs during class time! Answer the following questions about the experience.
   - How did you find yourself compensating for the hearing loss? Turning up the TV or radio? Asking others to write out information? Staying away from others? Getting angry or frustrated?
   - When you could not understand people, what did you do? Ask them to repeat? Ask them to speak louder? Answer even if you were unsure of what was said? Not respond at all?
   - If you answered when unsure, what was your response? Did you tend to agree or disagree with the speaker? Why?
   - What methods listed in the chapter were helpful? What other methods did you use to understand what was being said? Watching the speaker? Cupping your hand around ears?
   - How will this experience assist you when you care for a person with a hearing loss?

2. Cover your eyes with a blindfold so you cannot see. Keep the blindfold on for at least 1 hour as you go about your normal activities. Have someone act as a guide during this time. In addition to your normal activities, include the activities listed. Answer the questions about the experience.
   - Go outside with your guide and cross a street.
   - Visit a store or restaurant with your guide.
   - Eat a simple snack or meal.
   - Go to the toilet, wash your hands, and comb your hair.
   - Have your guide take you to a public area, place you in a chair or on a bench, and leave you alone for 5 to 10 minutes.

NOTE: You may wish to carry out this exercise using the blindfold and using this alternate method. If you wear glasses, cover the lenses with a heavy coating of petroleum jelly. This will simulate the vision experienced by a person with cataracts. Answer the questions for both experiences.

- How did you feel when you were unable to see what was going on around you?
- What noises or other sensory stimulants did you notice?
- When you were crossing the street, how did you feel? Safe? Frightened?
- When you were in a public area, what did you notice? How did you feel? How did others respond to you?
- How comfortable did you feel about eating when you could not see the food? How were you able to locate the food? What problems did you have?
- How did you manage in the bathroom? Were you able to find the equipment you needed? How competent did you feel about carrying out hand washing and grooming without seeing?
- What were your feelings when left alone in a public area for 5 to 10 minutes? How long did it *seem* to be before your guide returned? What concerns did you have? Safety? Fear of injury? Desertion?
- How will this experience assist you when caring for a person with a vision loss?

3. Have a group discussion with your classmates who have carried out the exercises to simulate vision and hearing problems. Answer these questions.
   - Which disability did you find the most difficult to tolerate? Why?
   - If you had to live with one of these disabilities, which one would you choose? Why?
   - What happened during these exercises that surprised you about being unable to see or hear? How does this discovery change your attitude about the disabilities?

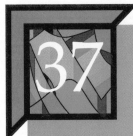

Caring for Mothers, Infants, and Children

Circle the Correct Answer

1. Which of these statements is *not true* about cloth diapers?
   a. When soiled, they are placed in the garbage
   b. They can be washed, dried, folded, and reused
   c. They are cheaper to use than disposable diapers
   d. Cloth diapers are available with Velcro fasteners

2. How do you remove formula from nipples?
   a. Place them in the sterilizer
   b. Squeeze hot, soapy water through the nipples
   c. Clean with a bottle brush
   d. Wash with cool, clean water

3. Which of the following must be reported to the nurse immediately?
   a. The baby "spits up" during burping
   b. The baby's bowel movement consists of hard, formed stool
   c. The baby's umbilical stump is dry
   d. The baby stops crying when picked up and cuddled

4. A sign of infection in the cord stump would be:
   a. A dried, blackened piece of tissue
   b. Redness or odour at the site
   c. Slight bleeding when the stump falls off
   d. Softening around the base of the cord

5. When a baby boy is circumcised, which of the following is *false?*
   a. the penis will look red, swollen, and sore.
   b. urination should be normal.
   c. the area will completely heal in 4 to 6 days.
   d. the penis should be cleaned with each diaper change.

6. When cleaning the circumcision, what is applied to prevent the penis from sticking to the diaper?
   a. Alcohol
   b. Soap and water
   c. Powder
   d. Petroleum jelly

7. What part of the body is cleaned with cotton swabs during the sponge bath?
   a. Nostrils
   b. Eyes
   c. Ears
   d. Cotton swabs are not used in any area

8. Which of the following indicates an infection in a postpartum woman?
   a. Dark red discharge 3 to 4 days after delivery
   b. An increase of lochia flow with activity
   c. A foul-smelling lochia
   d. Lochia alba that continues for 2 to 6 weeks after delivery

Fill-In-the-Blanks

9. Why is it important to respond to the cries of the baby or to feed the baby when he/she is hungry?

   _____

10. What can you do to prevent injury if you are changing a baby on a table or sofa?

    _____

11. What signs and symptoms would tell you that the infant may be ill?

    a. _____

    b. _____

    c. _____

    d. _____

    e. _____

    f. _____

    g. _____

    h. _____

    i. _____

    j. _____

    k. _____

    l. _____

    m. _____

12. What ways would be helpful to assist a mother with breastfeeding?

    a. _____

    b. _____

    c. _____

    d. _____

    e. _____

    f. _____

    g. _____

    h. _____

    i. _____

13. What are three forms of baby formula and how would you prepare each?

    a. _____

    b. _____

    c. _____

14. What measures are important to follow when a baby is bottle-fed?

    a. _____

    b. _____

    c. _____

    d. _____

    e. _____

    f. _____

    g. _____

    h. _____

    i. _____

15. What does it mean when it is said a baby is "fed on demand?"

    _____

16. How are bottles and other equipment cleaned to reduce the chance of infection?

    _____

17. What are two methods of burping a baby?

    a. _____

    b. _____

18. What should you do if a baby has diarrhea?

    _____

    Why? _____

    _____

19. How should the genital area be cleaned if the baby has had a large bowel movement or has a rash?

_____

20. When using a cloth diaper, how should you fold it for a boy?

_____

For a girl?

_____

21. Cord care includes

a. _____

b. _____

c. _____

d. _____

e. _____

f. _____

22. What are health reasons that parents may choose to have a son circumcised?

_____

23. Why is it important to plan well when bathing a baby?

_____

24. What safety measures should be followed when bathing a baby?

a. _____

b. _____

c. _____

d. _____

25. When you are giving a tub bath, when is the head washed?

_____

26. Why is it important to keep baby's nails short?

_____

What is used to trim the nails?

_____

27. Why is it best to trim a baby's nails when he/she is sleeping?

_____

28. List the signs and symptoms of postpartum complications.

a. _____

b. _____

c. _____

d. _____

e. _____

f. _____

g. _____

h. _____

i. _____

j. _____

k. _____

29. The mother will have an abdominal incision if her baby is delivered by

_____.

True or False

*Circle **T** for true or **F** for false. Rewrite all false statements to make them true.*

30. **T   F**   Never leave a baby unattended or with a sibling in a tub of water.

_____

_____

31. **T   F**   Formula may be heated safely in a microwave.

_____

_____

32. **T   F**   Extra bottles of formula can be stored in the refrigerator and used within 24 hours.

_____

_____

33. **T   F**   Diapers are changed only when the baby has a bowel movement.

_____

_____

34. **T   F**   Disposable diapers can be flushed down the toilet when soiled.

_____

_____

35. **T   F**   The umbilical stump dries up and falls off in 7 to 10 days.

_____

_____

36. **T   F**   Umbilical stump care is given every time a bath is given.

_____

_____

37. **T   F**   The diaper is applied loosely while the circumcision is healing.

_____

_____

Independent Learning Activities

Talk with a friend or family member who has recently had a baby. Ask the following questions:

1. How did she care for the umbilical cord stump?
   - Were there any problems with the cord healing?
   - Did she know the signs of a problem?
   - How many days did it take for the stump to fall off?

2. If the baby was a boy, was he circumcised?
   - If so, how did the mother care for the penis?
   - Did she know the signs of a problem?

3. Did the mother breastfeed the baby?
   - What were her reasons for deciding to breastfeed?
   - If she breastfed, how long did she breastfeed?
   - What were the advantages of breastfeeding?
   - What were the disadvantages of breastfeeding?

4. Did the mother choose to bottle-feed the baby?
   - What were her reasons for deciding to bottle-feed?
   - What were the advantages of bottle-feeding?
   - What were the disadvantages of bottle-feeding?

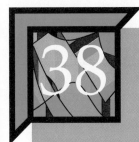

Developmental Disabilities

Fill-In-the-Blanks

1. What are some kinds of developmental disabilities?

   a. _____

   b. _____

   c. _____

   d. _____

   e. _____

   f. _____

   g. _____

2. What are some of the causes of intellectual disability?

   a. _____

   b. _____

   c. _____

   d. _____

   e. _____

   f. _____

3. If a mother develops rubella (German measles) during pregnancy, the baby may be

   _____.

4. What type of child abuse is a cause of intellectual disability?

   _____

5. The Canadian Association for Community Living believes the following:

   a. Children with an intellectual disability should

      live _____

      _____.

   b. Children with an intellectual disability should

      learn and play with _____

      _____.

   c. Adults with an intellectual disability should

      control their lives _____

      _____.

   d. Adults with an intellectual disability should live

      in a _____,

      _____,

      _____,

      and _____.

e. People with an intellectual disability have the right to privacy and to _____

_____ .

f. People with an intellectual disability should

learn about sex, _____ ,

_____ and other

_____ .

6. What are the physical characteristics of Down syndrome?

a. _____

b. _____

c. _____

d. _____

e. _____

f. _____

g. _____

7. What physical disorders or problems often affect children with Down syndrome?

a. _____

b. _____

c. At risk for _____

8. What therapies will be needed for children and adults with Down syndrome?

a. _____

b. _____

c. _____

d. _____

9. Infants at risk for cerebral palsy include

a. _____

b. _____

c. _____

d. _____

e. _____

f. _____

g. _____

h. _____

10. Lack of oxygen in early childhood can also cause cerebral palsy. The lack of oxygen can occur from

a. _____

b. _____

c. _____

d. _____

11. Describe the muscle movements of the three types of cerebral palsy.

a. Spastic

_____

b. Athetoid

_____

c. Ataxia

_____

12. What activities of daily living are affected because of spastic movements with cerebral palsy?

_____

13. What impairments may occur with cerebral palsy?

   a. _____

   b. _____

   c. _____

   d. _____

   e. _____

   f. _____

   g. _____

   h. _____

   i. _____

14. What functions are impaired with autism?

   a. _____

   b. _____

   c. _____

15. What behaviours would you expect to see in a person with autism?

   a. _____

   b. _____

   c. _____

   d. _____

   e. _____

   f. _____

   g. _____

   h. _____

   i. _____

   j. _____

   k. _____

   l. _____

   m. _____

   n. _____

   o. _____

16. What therapies are used to help the person with autism?

   a. _____

   b. _____

   c. _____

   d. _____

   e. _____

   f. _____

17. What kind of impairment can occur in these types of disability?

   a. Spina bifida occulta

   _____

   b. Meningocele

   _____

   c. Myelomeningocele

   _____

18. If the pressure inside the head of a child with hydrocephalus is not treated, what kinds of problems can result?

   a. _____

   b. _____

   c. _____

Matching

Match the types of spina bifida with the correct description.

19. _____ Part of spinal column is contained in a sac

20. _____ Spinal cord and nerves are usually normal; corrected with surgery

21. _____ Defect in vertebrae closure, but cannot be seen on outside of body

22. _____ Pouch contains nerves and spinal cord; loss of function below 22 of damage

a. Spina bifida occulta

b. Spina bifida cystica

c. Meningocele

d. Myelomenigocele

True or False

Circle **T** *for true or* **F** *for false. Rewrite all false statements to make them true.*

23. **T F** Mildly affected intellectually disabled people are slow to learn in school.

_____

_____

24. **T F** People with developmental disabilities do not develop reproductive organs or sexual urges.

_____

_____

25. **T F** All developmentally disabled people have the same amount of impairment.

_____

_____

26. **T F** Down syndrome causes some degree of intellectual disability in all affected people.

_____

_____

27. **T F** Cerebral palsy results from brain damage that occurs after birth.

_____

_____

28. **T F** Spastic cerebral palsy affects posture, balance, and movement.

_____

_____

29. **T F** Autism begins in early childhood.

_____

30. **T F** Autism can be cured with appropriate therapies.

_____

_____

31. **T F** Children with myelomeningocele may learn to walk using braces or crutches.

_____

_____

32. **T F** If a child has hydrocephalus, intellectual disabilities and neurological damage will occur without treatment.

_____

_____

Circle the Correct Answer

33. A person with epilepsy
    a. can never drive a car.
    b. may be able to function normally with medication.
    c. can never get a job.
    d. is intellectually disabled.

34. Hydrocephalus is treated by
    a. medications.
    b. closing the sac or pouch.
    c. placing a shunt in the brain.
    d. physical and occupational therapy.

Independent Learning Activities

Many communities have services available to families with children and adults who are developmentally disabled. Some communities have sheltered workshops, daycare, sheltered living centres, or physical and occupational therapy programs available. If your community has these services, ask permission to visit them and observe the people being served there. Answer these questions when you observe.

- What age groups are served in this program?
- What activities are available to the group?
- What training is required for the people who work there?
- How do the people in the program act? Happy? Bored? Withdrawn? Other reactions?

Assisting with Medications

Matching

Match the abbreviation with the meaning.

1. _____ By mouth   a. bid

2. _____ Per rectum   b. hs

3. _____ Every hour   c. npo

4. _____ Twice a day   d. po

5. _____ Every 2 hours   e. qid

6. _____ 4 times a day   f. pr

7. _____ Sublingual   g. qd

8. _____ Nothing by mouth   h. qh

9. _____ Hours of sleep   i. q2h

10. _____ Every day   j. sl

True or False

*Circle **T** for true or **F** for false. Rewrite all of the false statements to make them true.*

11. **T**   **F**   An elixir is medication dissolved in a concentrated sugar solution.

    _____

    _____

12. **T**   **F**   It is your responsibility to ensure your clients know about the side effects that can occur when taking their medications.

    _____

    _____

13. **T**   **F**   Part of your responsibility is to fill your client's pill box each week.

    _____

    _____

14. **T**   **F**   To make a suppository more comfortable for insertion, apply petroleum jelly to a suppository before handing it to the client.

    _____

    _____

15. **T** **F** A lozenge is a type of medication.

_____

_____

16. **T** **F** Some medications have to be taken on an empty stomach.

_____

_____

17. **T** **F** It is not in your scope of practice to sign MAR records.

_____

_____

18. **T** **F** Medication on transdermal disks absorbs over 24 hours.

_____

_____

19. **T** **F** You may purchase OTC medications for your client if requested to do so, as these are not prescription drugs.

_____

_____

20. **T** **F** Administering medications is beyond your scope of practice.

_____

_____

Fill-In-the-Blanks

21. Your role in assisting with medications may involve

a. _____

b. _____

c. _____

d. _____

e. _____

22. A side effect of a medication is

_____

_____

_____ .

23. Most MARs contain at least the following information:

a. _____

b. _____

c. _____

24. List and describe some of the routes that medication may be taken.

a. _____

b. _____

c. _____

d. _____

e. _____

25. Medications should be stored

    a. _____

    b. _____

    c. _____

    d. _____

    e. _____

26. The five "rights" of assisting with medications are

    a. _____

    _____

    b. _____

    _____

    c. _____

    _____

    d. _____

    _____

    e. _____

    _____

27. Medications come in many forms. List three and give an example of each.

    a. _____

    _____

    b. _____

    _____

    c. _____

    _____

28. If the medication is to dissolve under the person's tongue, you should

    a. _____

    b. _____

    c. _____

    d. _____

29. What information is on a prescription label?

    a. _____

    b. _____

    c. _____

    d. _____

    e. _____

    f. _____

    g. _____

    h. _____

Independent Learning Activities

1. Look through your medicine cabinet at home. Are any of the medications expired? Do you still need all of them?

2. If you have a prescription container, check to see if all of the required information is on the label.

3. Choose one medication you are familiar with, and look up the side effects. Did you realize that these side effects were possible?

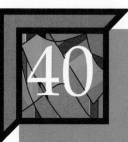

Measuring Height, Weight, and Vital Signs

Matching

The following words are used when discussing the pulse or blood pressure. Place "P" in front of words related to the pulse and "BP" in front of words related to the blood pressure.

1. _____ Radial

2. _____ Bradycardia

3. _____ Hypertension

4. _____ Systole

5. _____ Hypotension

6. _____ Diastole

7. _____ Apical

8. _____ Tachycardia

Match the site of the temperature to the normal range for that site.

	Site	Normal Range
9. _____	Oral	a. 35.5° to 37.5° C (95.9° to 99.5° F)
10. _____	Axillary	b. 34.7° to 37.3° C (94.5° to 99.1° F)
11. _____	Tympanic membrane	c. 35.8° to 38.0° C (94.6° to 100.4° F)

Circle the Correct Answer

12. Why is it important to keep a record of previous vital signs?
    a. So the support worker can prove that they were taken
    b. The doctor or nurse can compare each measurement
    c. The person's family can check to see if the care is being given
    d. The support worker can see if readings obtained are accurate as compared with others

13. When you take the vital signs and they have changed from a previous measurement, what should you do?
    a. Record the results promptly in the person's record
    b. Circle the changes in red
    c. Report the changes to the nurse promptly
    d. Take them again in 15 minutes

14. Which of these statements about electronic thermometers is *not true?*
    a. The temperature display is easily read
    b. If the probe is broken, the person could swallow mercury
    c. The temperature is rapidly measured
    d. Disposable covers reduce the possibility of spreading infection

15. If the person is smoking and you need to take an oral temperature, what should you do?
    a. Provide oral hygiene first
    b. Wait 20 minutes to take the temperature
    c. Take a rectal temperature instead
    d. Wait 45 minutes to take the temperature

16. For how long should you take an irregular pulse?
    a. 30 seconds
    b. 2 minutes
    c. 5 minutes
    d. 1 full minute

17. When assessing the pulse of an adult, which of the following pulse rates should be reported to the nurse immediately?
    a. 72
    b. 50
    c. 60
    d. 98

18. You are assigned to take blood pressures on several people. Which of these measurements should you report immediately?
    a. 140/80
    b. 138/90
    c. 150/110
    d. 96/70

Fill-In-the-Blanks

19. When would you expect vital signs to be measured?
    a. _____
    b. _____
    c. _____
    d. _____
    e. _____
    f. _____
    g. _____
    h. _____
    i. _____

20. The temperature should not be taken orally if the person
    a. _____
    b. _____
    c. _____
    d. _____
    e. _____
    f. _____
    g. _____
    h. _____

21. Where would you find the following pulses?
    a. Temporal
    _____
    b. Carotid
    _____
    c. Brachial
    _____
    d. Radial
    _____
    e. Femoral
    _____
    f. Popliteal
    _____
    g. Dorsalis pedis
    _____
    h. Apical
    _____

22. At what age would each of these pulse ranges be normal?

a. 80–180 _____

c. 70–110 _____

b. 80–120 _____

d. 60–100 _____

23. Where do you insert a tympanic membrane thermometer to measure body temperature?

_____

24. For how long is an axillary temperature taken with a glass thermometer?

_____

25 Why are the earpieces and diaphragm on a stethoscope cleaned with alcohol wipes before and after use?

_____

26. How can you prevent noise when you are using a stethoscope?

_____

27. What factors can affect the pulse rate?

a. _____

b. _____

c. _____

d. _____

e. _____

f. _____

g. _____

28. When you are measuring the pulse, what two characteristics of the pulse should be noted in addition to the rate?

_____

29. Why should you avoid using your thumb to take a pulse?

_____

30. Why do you keep your fingers or stethoscope in place after you count the pulse and while you count the respirations?

_____

31. How do these factors affect the blood pressure?

a. Age

_____

b. Gender

_____

c. Blood volume

_____

d. Stress

_____

e. Pain

_____

f. Exercise

_____

g. Weight

_____

h. Race

_____

i. Diet

_____

j. Drugs

_____

k. Position

_____

l. Smoking

_____

m. Alcohol

_____

32. If a person cannot stand up to have his/her height measured, what procedure will help you to gather this information?

_____

_____

_____

33. Why do you ensure your client has voided before you weigh him/her?

_____

_____

34. The height or length of a young child is taken from

the _____

_____ to the _____.

35. When you are taking blood pressures, what guidelines should you follow?

a. _____

b. _____

c. _____

d. _____

e. _____

f. _____

g. _____

h. _____

i. _____

j. _____

k. _____

l. _____

36. What is the normal respiratory rate for the following ages?

a. Newborn _____

b. 10 years _____

c. 2 years _____

d. Healthy adult _____

True or False

*Circle **T** for true or **F** for false. Rewrite all false statements to make them true.*

37. **T   F**   Glass thermometers can be cleaned and reused for several people.

_____

_____

38. **T   F**   Shake down the glass thermometer so the mercury is below the lines and numbers.

_____

_____

39. **T   F**   When you are storing a hand-held electronic thermometer, it is placed in a storage box.

_____

_____

40. **T   F**   To obtain the pulse deficit, subtract the apical pulse from the radial pulse.

_____

_____

Labelling

41. Name the parts of the stethoscope as indicated.

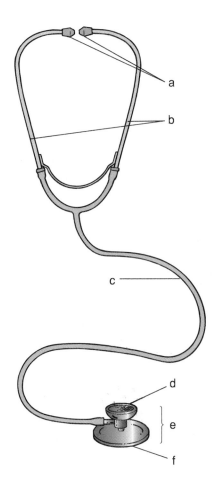

a. _____

b. _____

c. _____

d. _____

e. _____

f. _____

42. Fill in the drawings below so that the thermometers read correctly.
    a. 95.8° F   c. 100.2° F   e. 102.6° F   g. 36.5° C   i. 38.5° C
    b. 98.4° F   d. 101° F   f. 35.5° C   h. 37° C   j. 39.5° C

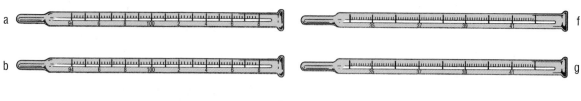

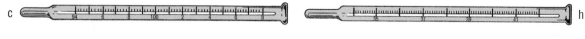

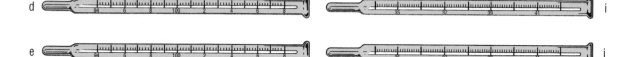

43. Fill in the following drawings so that the dials show the correct blood pressures.
    a. 168/102
    b. 104/68

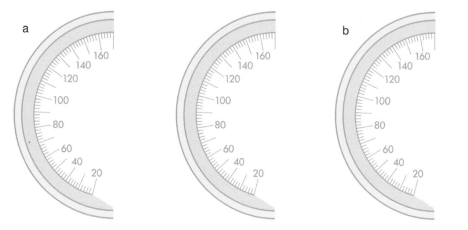

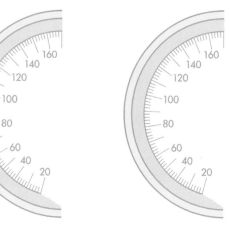

44. Fill in the following drawings so that the mercury columns show the correct blood pressure.
    a. 152/86
    b. 198/110

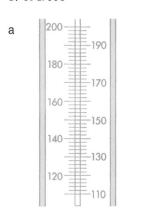
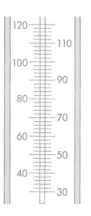
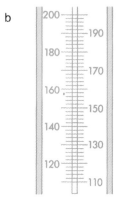
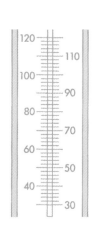

45. Record the temperatures shown.

   a. _____

   b. _____

   c. _____

Independent Learning Activities

1. Take turns measuring vital signs on three or four classmates. If possible, use a glass, electronic, and tympanic membrane thermometer for each person to see if there are any differences in temperatures. Write the results you get for each person.

   Use the table provided to keep a record of your readings. Answer the questions on the following page about this exercise.

Name	Temp	Pulse	Resp	B/P
	Glass	Radial	Rate	
	Elec		Rhythm	
	Tym		Depth	
	Glass	Radial	Rate	
	Elec		Rhythm	
	Tym		Depth	
	Glass	Radial	Rate	
	Elec		Rhythm	
	Tym		Depth	
	Glass	Radial	Rate	
	Elec		Rhythm	
	Tym		Depth	
	Glass	Radial	Rate	
	Elec		Rhythm	
	Tym		Depth	

- What type of thermometer was used? If different types of thermometers were used, how did the readings compare?
- What differences did you find in locating the radial pulse? The apical pulse?
- What differences did you find in the rate and rhythm of the pulses with various people?
- How were you able to measure the respirations so that the person was unaware you were doing it?
- What changes in respiration occurred if the person was aware you were counting?
- What differences in rhythm and depth of respirations did you observe with various people?
- How were you able to locate the correct spot to place the stethoscope diaphragm to take the blood pressure? What differences in this location did you find with various people?
- How did the sounds of the blood pressure differ among your classmates?
- What difficulties did you have with any of these measurements?
- What will you change about measuring vital signs on a person after this practice?

51. What are the functions of wound dressings?

    a. _____

    b. _____

    c. _____

    d. _____

    e. _____

52. Explain the method of applying tape to secure dressings.

    a. _____

    b. _____

53. What types of tape do not cause allergic reactions?

    _____

54. Why should you be careful to control nonverbal communication when changing a dressing?

    _____

55. How should you remove tape and old dressings from a wound?

    a. _____

    b. _____

56. Binders promote healing because they:

    a. _____

    b. _____

    c. _____

    d. _____

    e. _____

57. Explain when you would use each of these binders.

    a. Straight abdominal binder

    _____

    b. Breast binder

    _____

    c. T binders

    _____

58. How can you assist a person with a wound with the following concerns?

    a. Pain and discomfort

    _____

    b. Nutrition

    _____

    c. Infection

    _____

Circle the Correct Answer

59. Which of the following is a cause of skin breakdown?
    a. Good nutrition and hydration
    b. Decreased mobility
    c. Increased circulation
    d. Regular exercise program

60. What can you do to prevent skin tears on people you are caring for?
    a. Take daily baths
    b. Keep fingernails short and smoothly filed
    c. Wear jewellery with large stones
    d. Wear a clean uniform daily

61. To prevent pressure ulcers, the person may be placed on a surface such as
    a. a firm mattress.
    b. foam, air, alternating air, or gel mattresses.
    c. plastic or rubber material.
    d. a bed board.

62. Which of the following measures would not be helpful to prevent pressure ulcers?
    a. Apply moisturizer to dry areas such as hands, elbows, legs, ankles, and heels
    b. Reposition your client every four hours
    c. Massage well over reddened areas
    d. Keep heels off the bed

63. Which of the following measures would help to prevent stasis ulcers?
    a. Make sure clothing fits tightly
    b. Wear elastic stockings as ordered by doctor
    c. Massage any reddened area over pressure points
    d. Have person trim own toenails weekly

64. Montgomery ties are used to
    a. apply pressure to a wound.
    b. hold large dressings in place, especially if they must be changed frequently.
    c. cover drains in a wound.
    d. cover a wound when the person is allergic to adhesive tape.

65. Why may pain medication be given before a dressing change?
    a. To reduce discomfort during the dressing change
    b. To prevent the person from looking at the wound
    c. To prevent the person from seeing your non-verbal responses
    d. To prevent contamination of the wound

66. When removing an old dressing, it should be
    a. shown to the person.
    b. removed quickly from the wound with a quick pull.
    c. removed so that the soiled side is turned away from the person's sight.
    d. placed in the person's garbage can.

67. In second intention wound healing,
    a. the wound is cleaned and dead tissue is removed.
    b. sutures, staples, or adhesive strips hold the wound edges together.
    c. the wound is first left open and later closed with sutures.
    d. all of the above occur.

True or False

Circle T *for true or F for false. Rewrite all false statements to make them true.*

68. T F   When giving a back massage, massage the bony areas thoroughly.

_____

_____

69. T F   People sitting in a chair should be reminded to shift their weight every hour.

_____

_____

70. T F   When bathing or drying the person, rub vigorously.

_____

_____

71. T F   To prevent pressure ulcers, people who are incontinent should be checked frequently to prevent them from lying on wet linens.

_____

_____

72. T F   When applying tape, it should circle the entire body part to prevent swelling.

_____

_____

73. T F   Make sure you collect all equipment needed before you begin to change a non-sterile dressing.

_____

_____

74. T F   When changing a dressing, you should make sure that the person looks at his/her wound.

_____

_____

75. **T F** When changing a dressing, you only need to wear gloves if there is drainage.

_____

_____

Labelling

76. Place an X on five areas where pressure ulcers may form on a person lying in the supine position.

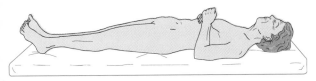

77. Place an X on six areas where pressure ulcers may form on a person lying in the lateral position.

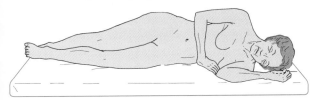

78. Place an X on six areas where pressure ulcers may form on a person lying in the prone position.

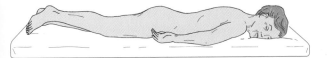

79. Place an X on three areas where pressure ulcers may form on a person lying in the Fowler's position.

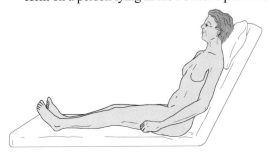

80. Place an X on four areas where pressure ulcers may form on a person in the sitting position.

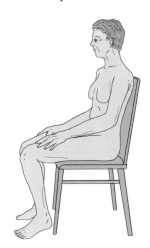

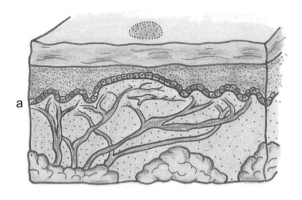

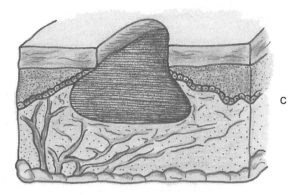

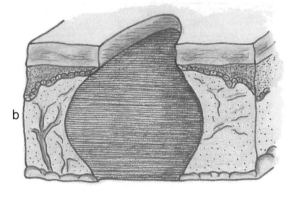

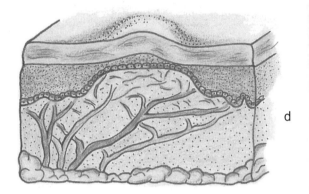

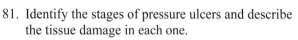

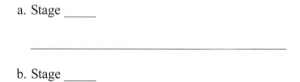

81. Identify the stages of pressure ulcers and describe the tissue damage in each one.

a. Stage _____

_____

b. Stage _____

_____

c. Stage _____

_____

d. Stage _____

_____

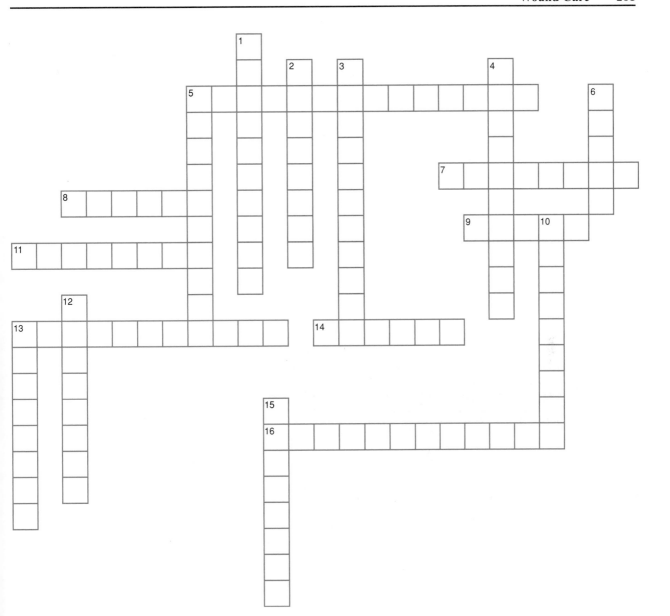

ACROSS

5. Pressure ulcer, pressure sore, bedsore *(2 words)*
7. Thick green, yellow, or brown discharge
8. Clear, watery drainage
9. Condition that results when there is not enough blood supply to organs and tissues
11. Condition where there is death of tissue
13. Thin, blood-tinged, watery drainage
14. Accident or violent act that injures the skin, mucous membranes, bones, and internal organs
16. Separation of wound along with protusion of abdominal organs

DOWN

1. Open wound with torn tissues and jagged edges
2. Partial-thickness wound caused by scraping away or rubbing of the skin
3. Open wound caused by poor blood return to the heart from the legs and feet *(2 words)*
4. Excessive loss of blood in a short period of time
5. Separation of wound layers
6. Break in the skin or mucous membranes
10. Closed wound caused by blow to the body
12. Open wound with clean, straight edges; usually intentionally produced with a sharp instrument
13. Break or rip in skin that separates the epidermis from the underlying tissues *(2 words)*
15. Collection of blood under the skin and tissues

Independent Learning Activities

Take turns with a classmate and carry out one or both of these exercises to understand how pressure ulcers may develop due to wrinkles or objects under a person. (It works best if the person wears thin clothes so the discomfort is more noticeable.)

a. Place a pencil on the seat of a chair and have a classmate sit on the pencil for 10 minutes. Keep time and remind the person not to move around to get more comfortable. Remember, many people cannot reposition themselves to relieve pressure.

b. Position a classmate in bed, making sure the bedclothes are wrinkled to form lumps under areas that may break down on a person. (For example, place the wrinkles under the coccyx in the supine position, or under the hip and shoulder in the side-lying position.) Make sure the person stays in the position for at least 10 minutes.

Answer these questions about the exercise.
- How long did it seem when you were left in one position for 10 minutes? Was it a short or long time to be uncomfortable?
- How many times did you try to reposition yourself?
- Were there any areas that felt sore after you were able to get up?
- How will this exercise affect your care of people in the future?

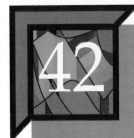

Heat and Cold Applications

Fill-In-the-Blanks

1. How does a heat application affect blood vessels?

   _____

2. How does dilation of the vessels help in healing?

   a. _____

   b. _____

3. Heat applications are used to:

   a. _____

   b. _____

   c. _____

   d. _____

   e. _____

4. What happens to blood vessels and blood flow when heat is applied for a long time?

   _____

5. What people or groups of people are at risk for burns from heat applications?

   a. _____

   b. _____

   c. _____

   d. _____

   e. _____

   f. _____

   g. _____

6. Which type of heat application is more penetrating—moist or dry?

   _____

7. How long may heat or cold be applied?

   _____

8. What type of soak is used to clean perineal or anal wounds?

   _____

9. When working in home care, what can be used to apply ice?

   a. _____

   b. _____

   c. _____

10. How often should you check the skin when cold compresses are in place?

    _____

11. What are the signs of complications when applying heat or cold?

   a. _____

   b. _____

   c. _____

   d. _____

   e. _____

   f. _____

   c. _____

   d. _____

   e. _____

   f. _____

   g. _____

   h. _____

   i. _____

   j. _____

   k. _____

12. What guideliness should be followed when you are applying heat or cold?

   a. _____

   b. _____

   l. _____

   m. _____

Matching

Match the types of heat applications with the correct definitions.

13. _____ Applications stay at desired temperature longer

14. _____ Does not penetrate deeply

15. _____ Temperature must be lower to prevent injury

16. _____ Heat penetrates deeper

17. _____ Higher temperature needed means burns are still a risk

18. _____ Moist heat applied to small area

19. _____ Water temperature should be hot (36.6° to 41.1° C)

20. _____ Tub may be used for applying moist heat to large area

   a. Dry heat

   b. Moist heat

   c. Compresses

   d. Soaks

Circle the Correct Answer

21. Which of these factors may make a person more susceptible to burns?
   a. Respiratory disorders
   b. Dehydration
   c. Circulatory disorders
   d. Infections

22. Heat should *not* be applied to which of these areas?
   a. Metal hip and knee replacements
   b. Joints
   c. Soft tissues
   d. Old fractures

23. A sitz bath may cause the person to feel weak or
faint because
   a. the bath increases pain in the area.
   b. blood flow increases in the pelvic area and less
   blood flows to other body parts.
   c. blood flow decreases in the pelvic area and
   more blood flows to other body parts.
   d. the person becomes chilled.

Independent Learning Activities

1. Role-play this situation with a classmate with each of you taking a turn as the person receiving a heat application to a body part. Answer the questions about the procedure and your feelings about having the heat applied to you.

   SITUATION: Mr. Singh is 45 and has an inflammation in his right calf. The nurse instructs you to apply moist, hot compresses to his leg.
   - What was Mr. Singh told about the procedure before the heat was applied to his leg?
   - How did you determine that the compress was the correct temperature?
   - What method did you use to keep the compress warm while it was on the leg?
   - What was used to cover the compress?
   - How often was the area checked while the compress was in place? When the area was checked, what signs and symptoms were observed?
   - What signs or symptoms would cause you to remove the compress and notify the nurse?
   - When you were acting as Mr. Singh, how did the compress feel? What were you asked about your comfort?
   - How warm did the compress feel at the end of 20 minutes? How warm was the skin in the area?

2. Role-play this situation with a classmate with each of you taking a turn as the person receiving a cold application to a body part. Answer the questions about the procedure and your feelings about having the cold applied to you.

   SITUATION: Mrs. Rosatti is 83. This morning she twisted her ankle going to the bathroom. The nurse instructs you to apply an ice bag to the area.
   - How will you prepare the ice bag? Why is it important to remove excess air?
   - How would you protect the skin from injury? Why is this important?
   - How will you secure the ice bag in place?
   - How often should you check the area? What signs and symptoms would you be observing? What response would cause you to remove the bag?
   - What would you tell Mrs. Rosatti when she asks why the ice must be removed after 20 minutes?
   - When you were acting as Mrs. Rosatti, how did the ice bag feel? What were you asked about your comfort?

Oxygen Needs

Fill-In-the-Blanks

1. What are the three processes that respiratory system function involves?

   a. _____

   b. _____

   c. _____

2. Explain how these factors affect oxygen needs.

   a. Respiratory system

   _____

   b. Cardiovascular system

   _____

   c. Red blood cell count

   _____

   d. Nervous system

   _____

   e. Aging

   _____

   f. Exercise

   _____

g. Fever

_____

h. Pain

_____

i. Drugs

_____

j. Smoking

_____

k. Allergies

_____

l. Pollutant exposure

_____

m. Nutrition

_____

n. Alcohol

_____

3. Hypoxia is a

   _____.

   What signs and symptoms would tell you the person has hypoxia?

   a. _____

   b. _____

   c. _____

   d. _____

   e. _____

   f. _____

   g. _____

   h. _____

   i. _____

   j. _____

   k. _____

   l. _____

   m. _____

   n. _____

   o. _____

4. What should you do if the person is wearing dark nail polish when you want to use the pulse oximeter?

   _____

5. When a pulse oximeter is used, what should be reported and recorded?

   a. _____

   b. _____

   c. _____

   d. _____

   e. _____

6. Why are gloves worn when collecting a sputum specimen?

   _____

7. Coughing and deep-breathing exercises help to prevent _____

   and _____.

8. How is the person instructed to exhale during cough and deep-breathing exercises?

   _____

9. Describe each of these oxygen sources.

   a. Wall outlet

   _____

   b. Oxygen tank

   _____

   c. Oxygen concentrator

   _____

11. Describe the following devices used to deliver oxygen.

   a. Simple face mask

   _____

   b. Partial-rebreather mask

   _____

   c. Nonrebreather mask

   _____

   d. Venturi mask

   _____

11. What should you do if the oxygen humidifier is bubbling?

   _____

12. What rules should you follow when handling the tubing for oxygen administration?

   a. _____

   b. _____

   c. _____

13. What fire safety rules should be followed if oxygen is in use?

   a. _____

   b. _____

   c. _____

   d. _____

   e. _____

   f. _____

   g. _____

   h. _____

14. If you observe that the oxygen rate is not set at the rate the nurse stated, what should you do?

   _____

15. Where should the support worker check for signs of irritation from the oxygen cannula or mask?

   _____

16. Why is a humidifier often used in oxygen administration?

   _____

17. Describe devices used when an artificial airway is needed.

   a. Oropharyngeal airway

   _____

   b. Nasopharyngeal airway

   _____

   c. Endotracheal tube

   _____

   d. Tracheostomy tube

   _____

18. How can you assist the nurse in caring for persons with artificial airways?

   a. _____

   b. _____

   c. _____

   d. _____

19. How can the person with an artificial airway communicate with you?

   _____

   _____

20. What are the parts of a tracheostomy tube?

   a. _____

   b. _____

   c. _____

21. When you are caring for a person with a tracheostomy, you should call the nurse if:

   a. _____

   b. _____

22. What measures are important to prevent aspiration with a tracheostomy?

   a. _____

   b. _____

   c. _____

   d. _____

   e. _____

f. _____

g. _____

23. When assisting with suctioning, the support worker may check the person's pulse, respirations, and

    pulse oximeter _____,

    _____, and

    _____ the procedure.

24. When the support worker is assisting with suctioning, the following should be reported to the nurse.

    a. _____

    b. _____

    c. _____

    d. _____

    e. _____

25. An Ambu bag is used to

    _____

    to prevent or treat hypoxia.

26. Why is it important to keep the call bell within reach and answer it promptly when you are caring for a person with mechanical ventilation?

    _____

    _____

27. When caring for a person with chest tubes, what information should be observed and reported to the nurse?

    a. _____

    b. _____

    c. _____

    d. _____

    e. _____

    f. _____

28. If you are caring for a person with chest tubes, what should you do if a chest tube comes out, after calling for help?

    a.

    _____

    b. _____

Matching

Match the tests with the correct description.

29. _____ Measures amount of air moving in and out of lungs

30. _____ Allows doctor to inspect trachea and bronchi

31. _____ Punctures and aspirates air or fluid from the pleura

32. _____ Evaluates changes in lungs

33. _____ Radioactive gas inhaled allows physician to see what areas are not getting air or blood

34. _____ Lab test measures amount of oxygen in the blood

a. Chest x-ray

b. Lung scan

c. Bronchoscopy

d. Thoracentesis

e. Pulmonary function tests

f. Arterial blood gases

Circle the Correct Answer

35. A pulse oximeter is used to measure
    a. oxygen concentration in arterial blood.
    b. the pulse rate.
    c. oxygen concentration in the lungs.
    d. amount of oxygen in the blood.

36. Which of these procedures may be done by a support worker?
    a. Administering oxygen therapy
    b. Suctioning
    c. Collecting a sputum specimen
    d. Performing tracheostomy care

37. When is the best time to collect a sputum specimen?
    a. At mealtime
    b. Early in the morning
    c. At bedtime
    d. After using mouthwash

38. What position is often preferred by people with difficulty breathing?
    a. Laying on one side
    b. Supine position
    c. Orthopneic position
    d. Prone position

39. Which of these statements is true about administering oxygen with a face mask?
    a. It irritates the nose and throat
    b. It makes talking difficult
    c. The person may eat and drink while it is in place
    d. Smoking is allowed in the room where the person is sitting

40. If the support worker is allowed to set up the oxygen administration system, which of the following would *not* be allowed?
    a. Collect oxygen administration device with the connecting tube
    b. Attach flow meter to wall outlet
    c. Attach humidifier to bottom of flow meter
    d. Apply oxygen administration device on the person

41. When the nurse is giving tracheostomy care, the support worker may be asked to assist when the ties are removed by
    a. holding the inner cannula in place.
    b. cleaning the outer cannula.
    c. cleaning the stoma.
    d. suctioning the tracheostomy.

42. Which of the following would be the responsibility of the support worker with a person on a mechanical ventilator?
    a. Reset the alarm if it rings
    b. Use established hand or eye signals for "yes" and "no"
    c. Listen carefully when the person tells what he/she needs
    d. Both b and c are correct

True or False

Circle **T** *for true or* **F** *for false. Rewrite all false statements to make them true.*

43. **T   F**   The sensor for the pulse oximeter is only used on the fingers.

   _____

   _____

44. **T   F**   The doctor must order oxygen because oxygen is a drug.

   _____

   _____

45. **T   F**   The support worker is responsible for administering oxygen.

   _____

   _____

46. **T   F**   The type of device used to deliver oxygen is decided by the nurse.

   _____

   _____

47. **T   F**   You may remove the cannula or mask used to administer oxygen.

   _____

   _____

48. **T** **F** The oxygen flow is turned off when the person receiving oxygen is out of the room.

_____

_____

49. **T** **F** Frequent oral hygiene should be given when the person is receiving oxygen therapy.

_____

_____

50. **T** **F** All tracheostomy tubes have three parts.

_____

_____

51. **T** **F** A cover is placed over the tracheostomy tube when outside to prevent dust, insects, and other small particles from entering the stoma.

_____

_____

52. **T** **F** Suctioning the upper airway may be done through the mouth and pharynx or the nose and pharynx.

_____

_____

53. **T** **F** Suctioning the lower airway may be done through the mouth and pharynx or the nose and pharynx.

_____

_____

54. **T** **F** Sterile technique is not required for oropharyngeal suctioning.

_____

_____

55. **T** **F** You may change the settings on a mechanical ventilator as needed.

_____

_____

56. **T** **F** When caring for a person with chest tubes, the drainage system is kept above the level of the person's chest.

_____

_____

57. **T** **F** Petrolatum gauze is kept at the bedside to cover the insertion site if a chest tube comes out.

_____

_____

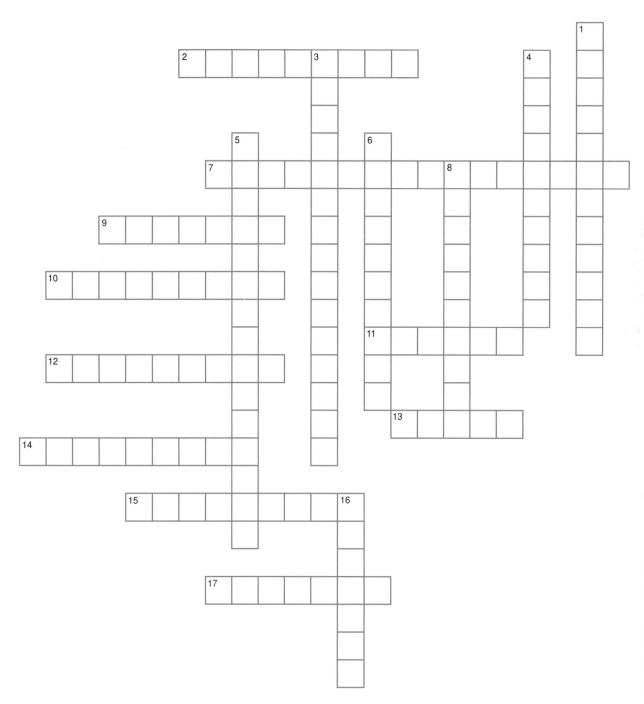

ACROSS

2. Rapid breathing; respirations are usually more than 24 per minute
7. Respirations that are rapid and deeper than normal
9. Process of withdrawing or sucking up fluids (secretions)
10. Slow breathing; respirations are fewer than 10 per minute
11. Expectorated mucus
12. Reduced amount of oxygen in the blood
13. Lack or absence of breathing
14. Harmful chemical or substance in the air or water
15. Being able to breathe deeply and comfortably only while sitting or standing
17. Difficult, laboured, or painful breathing

DOWN

1. Collection of air in the pleural space
3. Escape and collection of fluid in the pleural space *(2 words)*
4. Collection of blood in the pleural space
5. Respirations that are slow, shallow, and sometimes irregular
6. Bloody sputum
8. Process of inserting an artificial airway
16. Sensitivity to a substance that causes the body to react with signs and symptoms

Independent Learning Activities

1. This activity will help you to understand how a person feels when she or he has breathing problems.
   - Have a classmate count your respirations while you are resting (the resting rate).
   - Exercise (run or jog in place, do situps, etc.) for at least 2 minutes.
   - What differences do you notice when you inhale? When you exhale?

2. Have a classmate count your respirations as soon as you complete this activity. Compare this number to your resting rate.
   - Were you breathing with your mouth closed or open?
   - What differences did you note in your breathing?
   - How long did it take for your rate to return to the resting rate?
   - How do you think this activity relates to a person who has breathing problems?

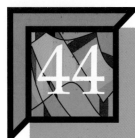

Assisting with the Physical Examination

Matching

Match the descriptions with the correct position.

1. _____ Hips down to edge of table, knees flexed, feet in stirrups   a. Supine

2. _____ Lying on side with upper leg flexed   b. Lithotomy

3. _____ Lying on back with legs together or knees flexed   c. Knee-chest

4. _____ Kneeling with body supported on knees and chest   d. Sims'

Fill-In-the-Blanks

5. What should you explain to the person about the positions used in the examination?

   a. _____

   b. _____

   c. _____

   d. _____

6. Why is the person asked to urinate before an examination?

   a. _____

   b. _____

7. Why is it important to cover a person with a drape during an examination?

   _____

8. Why should a female support worker stay in the examination room with a female being examined by a male doctor?

   a. _____

   b. _____

9. When a child is being examined, what are two reasons parents may remain in the room?

   a. _____

   b. _____

10. What needs to be done to the examination area
after an examination is completed?

a. Discard

_____

b. Replace

_____

c. Clean

_____

d. Label and send

_____

Labelling

11. Label each of the examination instruments. What
is the use of each instrument?

a. _____

b. _____

c. _____

d. _____

e. _____

f. _____

g. _____

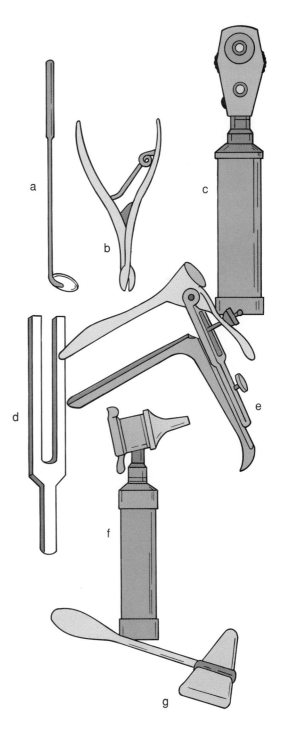

Independent Learning Activities

You probably have had a physical examination at some time. It is likely that you needed one to be a student in this class. Answer these questions concerning your own experience with physical examinations.

- Who explained to you what to expect during the examination? What were you told about any discomfort? Positioning? Lack of privacy?
- What steps were taken to give you privacy? While you changed clothes? During the examination?
- Who was present during the examination? Were you given a choice of having a person with you while the doctor examined you? How did you feel about having (or not having) another person in the room?
- How did you know what was going to be done next? Was each step explained to you?
- What questions were you able to ask? Who was available to answer any questions? Did you feel as if your questions were answered so that you understood?
- How did the doctor or nurse make you feel when you asked a question? As if they cared about giving you an answer you could understand? As if you were bothering them?
- How were you positioned during the examination? Which position in the textbook was used? How did you feel in the position? How long did you need to stay in the position?
- How does this experience help you to understand the feelings of people you may assist during a physical examination?

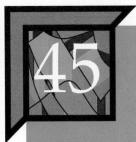

The Patient Having Surgery

Matching

Match the descriptions or examples given with the correct type of surgery.

1. _____ Done immediately to save the person's life

2. _____ Type of surgery done when the coronary arteries are blocked

3. _____ Done for the person's well-being

4. _____ Type of surgery needed after an accident

5. _____ Must be done soon to prevent further damage or disease

6. _____ Cosmetic surgery is an example of this type of surgery

a. Elective surgery

b. Emergency surgery

c. Urgent surgery

Determine when each of these events occur during the surgical process.

7. _____ Chest x-ray, CBC, and ECG

8. _____ Vital signs are measured every 15 minutes for first hour

9. _____ Coughing and deep breathing exercises as ordered

10. _____ Preoperative teaching

11. _____ Elastic stockings are applied

12. _____ Operative permit signed

a. Preoperatively

b. Postoperatively

Fill-In-the-Blanks

13. Who is responsible for telling the person and family about the need for surgery?

_____

14. What behaviours could indicate a person is fearful or concerned about surgery?

_____

15. What can you do to assist in the psychological care of the surgical patient?

    a. _____

    b. _____

    c. _____

    d. _____

    e. _____

    f. _____

16. What are fears the person may have about surgery?

    a. _____

    b. _____

    c. _____

    d. _____

    e. _____

    f. _____

    g. _____

    h. _____

    i. _____

    j. _____

    k. _____

    l. _____

17. The surgical patient may be concerned about situations such as:

    a. _____

    b. _____

    c. _____

    d. _____

    e. _____

18. What should you do if the person or family asks you the results of the surgery?

_____

19. Why is a person NPO 6 to 8 hours before surgery?

_____

20. You should report any loose teeth a child has pre-operatively because _____

_____.

21. Children can be prepared for surgery by using

_____

_____.

22. Children are often afraid to leave their parents when they go to surgery. Some hospitals allow a parent to _____

_____.

23. Why is the following personal care done before surgery?

    a. Bath and shampoo

    _____

    b. Make-up and nail polish removed

    _____

c. Cap on hair

_____

_____

d. Oral hygiene

_____

_____

24. When giving personal care to hair, what needs to be done before a surgical cap is put on the person?

_____

_____

25. Do not allow the person to _____

_____

during oral hygiene before surgery.

26. What valuables are removed for safekeeping during surgery?

_____

_____

27. How do you know where the valuables are located so you can find them after surgery?

_____

_____

28. What should be done if a person tells you he/she wants to wear a wedding band or religious medal during surgery?

_____

_____

29. A skin prep before surgery reduces

_____

that can cause an infection.

30. When a skin prep is done, the _____

and a _____ are prepped.

31. When doing a skin prep, you should shave in which direction?

_____

_____

32. Why is it important to be very careful not to cut, scratch, or nick the skin during a skin prep?

_____

_____

33. When a person receives a preoperative medication, he/she is at risk for falls and accidents because the medications can cause

_____

_____

34. How can you help to protect the person from injury when preoperative medications are given?

a. _____

b. _____

c. _____

d. _____

e. _____

35. What type of anesthesia produces loss of sensation in a large area of the body?

_____

_____

36. What equipment should be placed in the person's room for use when he/she returns from surgery?

a. _____

b. _____

c. _____

d. _____

e. _____

f. _____

37. How would you prepare the patient's bed and other furniture for his/her return from surgery?

    a. _____

    b. _____

    c. _____

    d. _____

38. Why is the person repositioned every 1 to 2 hours after surgery?

    _____

39. Why are leg exercises important postoperatively?

    _____

40. What postoperative observations are important?

    a. _____

    b. _____

    c. _____

    d. _____

    e. _____

    f. _____

    g. _____

    h. _____

41. Coughing, deep breathing, and incentive spirometry are very important for postoperative patients. Why is it especially important for older people?

    _____

42. What complications can be prevented with early ambulation?

    _____

43. Before ambulating a person after surgery, what steps should you take to prevent injury?

    a. _____

    b. _____

44. What is the reason a person may be NPO after surgery?

    _____

45. While a person is NPO, how are fluids given?

    _____

    What can you do to keep the person comfortable while he/she is NPO?

    _____

46. Why is it important to report that a person has voided 8 hours after surgery?

    _____

47. What factors can cause pain after surgery?

    a. _____

    b. _____

    c. _____

    d. _____

48. Personal hygiene after surgery is especially important because:

    a. _____

    b. _____

    c. _____

25. What is the major sign of cardiac arrest?
    a. No pulse
    b. Low blood pressure
    c. Hemorrhage
    d. Flushed, warm skin

26. When should you begin CPR?
    a. When a person loses consciousness
    b. When breathing has ceased
    c. As soon as you find the person
    d. When you have determined there is no pulse and no breathing

27. When you find a person who is unresponsive, when should you activate the EMS system?
    a. As soon as you determine that the person is unresponsive
    b. After you have determined breathlessness
    c. After you have determined pulselessness
    d. After performing CPR for 1 full minute

28. Which of the following should be done during mouth-to-mouth resuscitation to an adult?
    a. Pinch the nostrils
    b. Breathe into the person's nostrils and mouth at the same time
    c. Keep the person's chin down toward the chest
    d. Give chest compressions and breaths at the same time

29. Where should you position yourself when doing chest compressions with CPR?
    a. At the person's head
    b. Straddling the person's legs
    c. With your shoulders directly over the chest
    d. At the side of the person with your elbows bent

30. What is the rate of compressions and rescue breaths done in one-rescuer CPR?
    a. 5 compressions and 1 ventilation
    b. 5 compressions and 2 ventilations
    c. 15 compressions and 1 ventilation
    d. 15 compressions and 2 ventilations

31. When giving chest compressions to a child younger than 8 years, the sternum should be depressed
    a. 2.5 to 4.0 cm.
    b. 1.3 to 2.5 cm.
    c. 4 to 5 cm.
    d. 5.0 to 7.6 cm.

32. What is the rate of chest compressions when giving CPR to an adult?
    a. 60 per minute
    b. 80 to 100 per minute
    c. 40 to 50 per minute
    d. One compression every 10 seconds

33. Which one the following steps would be used to prevent or treat shock?
    a. Set the person in a comfortable chair
    b. Expose the skin of the person to allow for cooling
    c. Control hemorrhage
    d. Turn the head to one side

34. Which of these steps would be correct if the person is having a seizure?
    a. Lay the person flat on the back
    b. Hold arms and legs still during the seizures
    c. Turn the head to one side
    d. Place a soft object between the teeth of the person

35. A partial-thickness burn
    a. is very painful.
    b. destroys nerve endings.
    c. injures or destroys the fat layer, muscle, and bone.
    d. is not very painful.

Emergency Responses

In this condition, the victim's signs and symptoms are:
- *Clutches at the throat*
- *Cannot breathe, speak, or cough*
- *Is pale and cyanotic*

36. What has occurred?

    _____

37. What actions should be taken?

    a. _____

    b. _____

In this condition, the victim's signs and symptoms are:
- *Low blood pressure*
- *Rapid and weak pulse*
- *Rapid respirations*
- *Cold, moist, and pale skin*
- *Confusion*
- *Bleeding*

38. What has occurred?

_____

39. What action should be taken?

    a. _____

    b. _____

    c. _____

    d. _____

    e. _____

In this condition, the signs and symptoms are:
- *Sweating*
- *Shortness of breath, dyspnea*
- *Respiratory congestion*
- *Swelling of the larynx*
- *Hoarseness*

40. What is the condition?

_____

41. What action should be taken?

    a. _____

    b. _____

    c. _____

    d. _____

Independent Learning Activities

1. Consider the following situation and answer the questions about how you would handle an emergency.

   SITUATION: You are eating lunch at a fast-food restaurant when a child at the next table begins to gasp for air. The mother cries out, "Jimmy is choking. Someone help me!"
   - How do you think you would react to a situation like this?
   - What would you say to Jimmy and his mother?
   - What would you do first?
   - How would you attempt to dislodge the object that is choking Jimmy?
   - What would you do to prevent contracting any infection from Jimmy? What equipment might be available in the restaurant that you could use?
   - How long would you continue to try to help Jimmy?

2. Consider how you would handle the following situation and answer the questions accordingly.

   SITUATION: As you attempt to remove the object obstructing Jimmy's breathing, he suddenly goes limp and is unresponsive.
   - How would you feel now that Jimmy is unresponsive?
   - What would you do first after he becomes unresponsive?
   - What would you want to check? How often?
   - What changes would you make in the procedure after he becomes unresponsive?
   - What concerns would you have now about infection control?
   - How long would you continue to help Jimmy?

3. Consider the following situation and answer the questions about what you would do if this emergency happened to you.

   SITUATION: You are shopping in a local discount store. As you turn a corner into the next aisle, you find an older man slumped against the shelves.
   - How would you feel about providing emergency care in this situation?
   - What concerns would you have about infection control? What could you do to decrease risk to yourself? What equipment might be available in the store that you could use?
   - What would be the first thing you would do?
   - How would you position the man?
   - What do you need to check first after repositioning the man?
   - If you find a pulse, but no respirations, what should you do?
   - If you find no pulse and no respirations, what should you do?
   - How long would you continue to provide emergency care to the man?

4. Consider the following situation and answer the questions about how you would handle this emergency.

   SITUATION: You are accompanying a group of 10-year-olds on a school trip to a nature preserve. Jeremy trips over a tree root and falls on a broken bottle. His arm is deeply cut and bright red blood is coming out of the wound in spurts. He is sitting on the ground crying and looks very pale. When you touch him, he is perspiring and feels cold.
   - How well do you think you would handle an emergency like this? What would be the most difficult part of helping this child?
   - What is the first thing you should do?
   - How can you best control the bleeding? What might be available to use if you were out in a nature preserve with a group of children?
   - How could you best protect the wound from contamination?
   - How could you protect yourself from blood-borne pathogens?
   - What do his symptoms (pale, cool, perspiring) tell you? How would you help to treat this problem?

Medical Terminology

Matching

Match the word in Column A with the correct definition in Column B.

Column A

1. _____ Neuralgia
2. _____ Gastrotomy
3. _____ Cholecystectomy
4. _____ Dysuria
5. _____ Gastritis
6. _____ Enteritis
7. _____ Bacteriogenic
8. _____ Glossitis
9. _____ Cyanotic
10. _____ Dermatology
11. _____ Oophorectomy
12. _____ Colostomy
13. _____ Nephritis
14. _____ Bronchoscope
15. _____ Proctoscopy

Column B

a. Painful or difficult urination

b. Inflammation of kidneys

c. Bluish colour

d. Caused by bacteria

e. Study of the skin

f. Incision into large intestine

g. Instrument used to examine bronchi

h. Inflammation of the tongue

i. Nerve pain

j. Examination of rectum with instrument

k. Excision of gallbladder

l. Excision of ovary

m. Incision into stomach

n. Inflammation of stomach

o. Inflammation of intestine

Definitions

Write the definition of each prefix in the space provided.

16. auto-_____

17. brady-_____

18. circum-_____

19. dys-_____

20. ecto-_____

21. leuk-_____

22. macro-_____

23. neo-_____

24. supra-_____

25. uni-_____

Write the definition of each suffix in the space provided.

36. -asis_____

37. -genic_____

38. -ism_____

39. -oma_____

40. -phasia_____

41. -ptosis_____

42. -plegia_____

43. -megaly_____

44. -scopy_____

45. -stasis_____

Write the definition of each root word in the space provided.

26. adeno_____

27. angio_____

28. broncho_____

29. cranio_____

30. duodeno_____

31. entero_____

32. gyneco_____

33. masto_____

34. myelo_____

35. pyo_____

Write the correct abbreviations for the following phrases or terms.

46. Abdomen _____

47. Before meals _____

48. After meals _____

49. With _____

50. Cancer _____

51. Discontinued _____

52. Lower left quadrant _____

53. Every day _____

54. Range of motion _____

Word Search

Identify the abbreviations in questions 55 through 80 and write the word in the space. Find the words in the following puzzle.

55. $\overline{s}$ _____

56. am _____

57. CA _____

58. H_2O _____

59. q _____

60. wt _____

61. ht _____

62. w/c _____

63. $\overline{c}$ _____

64. stat _____

65. O_2 _____

66. abd _____

67. CVA _____

68. Twice a day _____

69. Complete bed rest _____

70. Nothing by mouth _____

71. When necessary _____

72. Every night at bedtime _____

73. Range of motion _____

74. Right lower quadrant _____

75. Soap suds enema _____

76. Three times a day _____

77. Four times a day _____

78. Every other day _____

79. Left lower quadrant _____

80. Vital signs _____

N	E	U	N	I	T	N	O	C	S	I	D	R	O	E	S	S
U	S	R	P	R	N	A	Q	O	A	W	I	T	H	O	U	T
R	T	I	O	N	E	M	O	D	B	A	B	E	E	Q	L	R
S	A	M	L	O	C	C	D	A	H	H	E	I	G	H	T	O
E	T	B	U	T	A	L	L	C	O	R	V	W	E	L	L	K
M	O	R	N	I	N	G	L	Q	B	W	E	I	G	H	T	E
C	X	R	I	D	C	E	M	I	A	R	R	T	Q	L	L	V
A	Y	W	A	T	E	R	H	E	A	R	Y	H	I	I	C	E
R	G	R	A	H	R	G	R	A	M	V	S	S	E	E	D	R
E	E	L	W	E	L	I	M	M	E	D	I	A	T	E	L	Y
E	N	C	O	U	R	A	G	E	M	E	N	T	F	E	E	L

Circle the Correct Answer

Circle the word in each group that is spelled correctly.

81. Slow heart rate
    a. Bradecardia
    b. Bradycardia
    c. Bradacordia
    d. Bradicardia

82. Difficulty in urinating
    a. Dysuria
    b. Dysurya
    c. Dysuira
    d. Disuria

83. Paralysis on one side of the body
    a. Hemyplegia
    b. Hemaplegia
    c. Hemoplega
    d. Hemiplegia

84. Opening into the ileum
    a. Illeostomy
    b. Ileostomy
    c. Ileastoma
    d. Illiostomy

85. Blue colour or condition
    a. Cyonosis
    b. Cyinosis
    c. Cyanosis
    d. Cianosys

86. Opening into trachea
    a. Tracheastomy
    b. Trachiostomy
    c. Tracheostome
    d. Tracheostomy

87. Pain in a nerve
    a. Neuralgia
    b. Neuroalgia
    c. Nourealgia
    d. Neurilegia

88. Examination of a joint with a scope
    a. Arthoscope
    b. Arthroscopy
    c. Arethroscopy
    d. Artheroscope

89. Rapid breathing
    a. Tachepnea
    b. Tachypinea
    c. Tachypnea
    d. Tachypnia

90. Removal of gallbladder
    a. Cholecystectomy
    b. Cholcystectomy
    c. Cholicystetomy
    d. Cholecistectomy

Using Word Elements

The following words are made up of prefixes, root words, and suffixes. Identify each of the word elements using one of these methods:

Circle the prefixes in black, the root words in red, and the suffixes in blue.

OR

Highlight the prefixes in yellow, the root words in pink, and the suffixes in blue.

In the space following each word, define the word.

91. Hepatomegaly _____

    _____

92. Hemiplegia _____

    _____

93. Cholecystectomy _____

    _____

94. Laparotomy _____

    _____

95. Bradycardia _____

    _____

96. Neuropathy _____

    _____

97. Tachypnea _____

    _____

98. Polyuria _____

    _____

99. Pyorrhea _____

103. Bronchoscopy _____

_____

_____

100. Dysphagia _____

104. Encephalopathy _____

_____

_____

101. Erythrocytopenia _____

105. Stomatitis _____

_____

_____

102. Leukocyte _____

_____

Independent Learning Activities

1. Medical terms are found in magazines, newspapers, and books. After studying this chapter, you should be able to identify and define these terms. Try the following exercises to practise using this knowledge every day, not just in class.
   - Go to the library and look at the health section of a newspaper. Look up articles in this section and write down any words you do not understand. Compare these words with the terms and word parts you have learned in this chapter. How many can you define?
   - Many popular magazines have a section on health, medicines, and diseases. Look at three or four magazines in the library and see how many medical terms are used. Write down the terms that you find. How many of these were you able to define?

2. The next time you or a member of your family visits the doctor and is instructed to fill a prescription, look at what the doctor has written. Do you see any abbreviations that you learned in this chapter? What do they mean? How did this chapter help you to understand what was written?

3. Make flash cards of the prefixes, suffixes, and root words in Chapter 48. Put the meaning of each one on the back of the appropriate card. Work alone or with a partner and, by looking at the cards, practise identifying the correct meaning of each term.

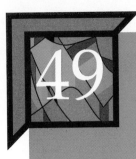

49

Your Job Search

True or False

Circle **T** *for true or* **F** *for false. Rewrite all false statements to make them true.*

1. **T F** The longer your résumé is the better.

_____

_____

2. **T F** A letter of application is also called a cover letter.

_____

_____

3. **T F** Your cover letter should be at least two pages long.

_____

_____

4. **T F** If you e-mail your letter and résumé, it is a good idea to also deliver a hard copy.

_____

_____

5. **T F** Admit to your prospective employer if you have been fired from a previous job.

_____

_____

6. **T F** When filling out a job application, you may skip parts that are unimportant to you.

_____

_____

7. **T F** Asking people you know about possible jobs at their workplace is not a good way to find a job.

_____

_____

8. **T F** An employer is not as concerned about your dependability as he/she may be about your job skills.

_____

_____

9. **T F** If you were fired from a previous job, it is alright to write on a job application that you resigned.

_____

_____

10. **T   F**   When you are being interviewed for a job, it is acceptable to ask about starting salary, work hours, and new employee orientation.

_____

_____

Circle the Correct Answer

11. When going to an interview, it would be appropriate to
    a. have a glass of wine before arriving to relax you.
    b. wear a sweatsuit and athletic shoes to show that you are physically fit.
    c. avoid wearing heavy perfume or after-shave lotion.
    d. arrive exactly at the time of the interview so you do not have time to get nervous.

12. After a job interview, you should
    a. thank the interviewer.
    b. state that you look forward to hearing from him or her.
    c. write a thank-you note.
    d. do all of the above.

Fill-In-the-Blanks

13. Describe the two basic résumé styles.

    a. _____

    _____

    b. _____

    _____

14. As you write your résumé, what questions should you ask yourself?

    a. _____

    b. _____

    c. _____

    d. _____

    e. _____

15. What are some sources to help in your job search?

    a. _____

    b. _____

    c. _____

    d. _____

16. Your letter of application should include

    a. _____

    b. _____

    c. _____

    d. _____

    e. _____

17. In an interview, what is the employer looking for?

    a. _____

    b. _____

    c. _____

    d. _____

18. You can prepare for an interview by

    a. _____

    b. _____

    c. _____

    d. _____

19. You can do several things during the interview to help you get the job. Some of these are

    a. _____

    b. _____

    c. _____

    d. _____

e. _____

f. _____

20. Before accepting a job, find out

a. _____

b. _____

21. When you write a thank-you note after a job interview, what information should it include?

a. _____

b. _____

c. _____

Preparing to Work

The following questions will give you practice in filling out applications, preparing for interviews, and identifying how you will deal with day-to-day work. NOTE: Some of the answers may be found in the textbook, but many require you to answer for your individual situation.

22. These questions apply to filling out a job application. Use black ink and block printing when answering these questions. Make sure your writing is legible.
   a. How will you respond to a question on the application that does not apply to you?

   _____

   _____

   b. Why is the above action important?

   _____

   _____

   c. What information will you provide if you have been arrested and convicted of a felony?

   _____

   _____

d. How will you explain a gap in your employment history?

_____

_____

e. What reasons will you give about leaving previous jobs?

_____

_____

f. List three references you can use, including names, titles, addresses, and telephone numbers.

_____

_____

_____

g. Have you asked these people for permission to use them as references?

_____

_____

23. Look at the questions you have answered for question 22.

a. Have you been honest in answering them?

_____

b. Did you use black ink as directed?

_____

c. Did you use block print as directed?

_____

d. Is your printing legible?

_____

e. Why is it important that you followed directions and were honest?

_____

_____

24. Answer these questions about how you will prepare for a job interview.
   a. How can you make sure you will be on time for the interview?

   _____

   _____

   b. How will you travel to the interview?

   _____

   Is this transportation reliable? _____

   Do you have a backup plan? _____

   c. Choose an outfit to wear to the interview. Is it conservative and tasteful?

   _____

   Is it clean and well-maintained? _____

   Do you have an alternate outfit available in case you spill something at the last minute?

   _____

   d. What shoes will you wear? _____

   _____

   Do they need to be polished or repaired?

   _____

   e. What personal hygiene do you think is important before the interview?

   _____

   _____

   f. How do you plan to style your hair?

   _____

   What cosmetics will you use (make-up, cologne, after-shave, and so on)?

   _____

   g. What jewellery will you wear?

   _____

   h. When you arrive for the interview, what you say to the receptionist?

   _____

   i. Make a list of your skills that you can g the interviewer.

   _____

   _____

   _____

   _____

   _____

   _____

   _____

   _____

   _____

   j. How can you find out if you use good e tact and positive body language?

   _____

   Why is it important to know about these

   _____

25. How will you answer these questions if the viewer asks them?

   a. Tell me about yourself.

   _____

   _____

b. Please tell me about your career goals.

_____

_____

c. What are you doing currently to achieve these goals?

_____

_____

d. Describe what you consider to be *professional* behaviour.

_____

_____

e. Tell me about your last job.

_____

_____

f. What did you like most about your last job?

_____

Least?

_____

g. What would your supervisors and co-workers tell me about your dependability?

_____

_____

Your skills?

_____

Your ability to adapt?

_____

h. Of all your functions, which presented the most difficulty for you?

_____

i. How did you handle this difficulty?

_____

j. How do you set priorities?

_____

_____

k. In what ways have your past experiences prepared you for this position?

_____

_____

l. If there were one thing that you could change about your last job, what would it be?

_____

_____

m. How do you handle problems with clients and co-workers?

_____

_____

n. Why do you want to work here?

_____

o. Why should this agency hire you?

_____

26. Make a list of questions you may want to ask the interviewer.

a. _____

b. _____

c. _____

d. _____

e. _____

f. _____

g. _____

h. _____

i. _____

j. _____

27. Before you accept a job and begin to work, you need to answer these questions.
   a. Who will care for your child/children on a regular basis?

   _____

   b. What backup plan do you have if your babysitter is ill or unavailable?

   _____

   c. What plan do you have if a child becomes sick or injured while you are at work?

   _____

   d. What is your usual method of transporta[tion to] work?

   _____

   Is it always reliable?

   _____

   What backup plan do you have for transportation?

   _____

   _____

Independent Learning Activities

1. Why do you feel you will be a good support worker? What qualities and characteristics do you have tha[t] be helpful? How can you improve qualities and characteristics that you feel are weaknesses?

2. Have you ever applied for a job? How did you feel when you were being interviewed? After reading thi[s] chapter, in what ways could you improve future interviews?

3. How many agencies in your area employ support workers? What is a typical starting salary?

4. Who are three people you could use as references when applying for a job? Ask for permission to use th[ese] people as references. Make a list of these people and their titles, addresses, telephone numbers, and e-m[ail ad]dresses to use when you apply for a job.